THE LOW FODMAP DIET COOKBOOK

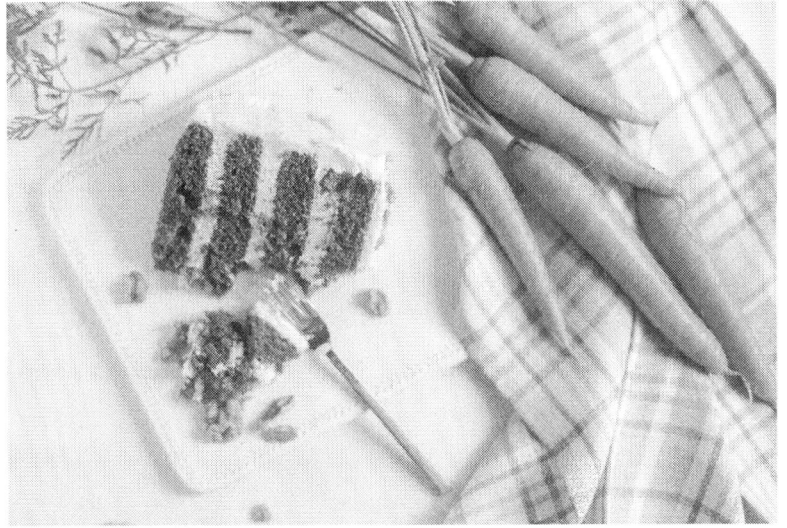

THIS RECIPE BOOK WILL HELP YOU TO FIND THE IBS SOLUTION, ELIMINATE DIGESTIVE DISORDERS, SOOTHE SYMPTOMS, AND KEEP YOUR GUT HEALTHY!

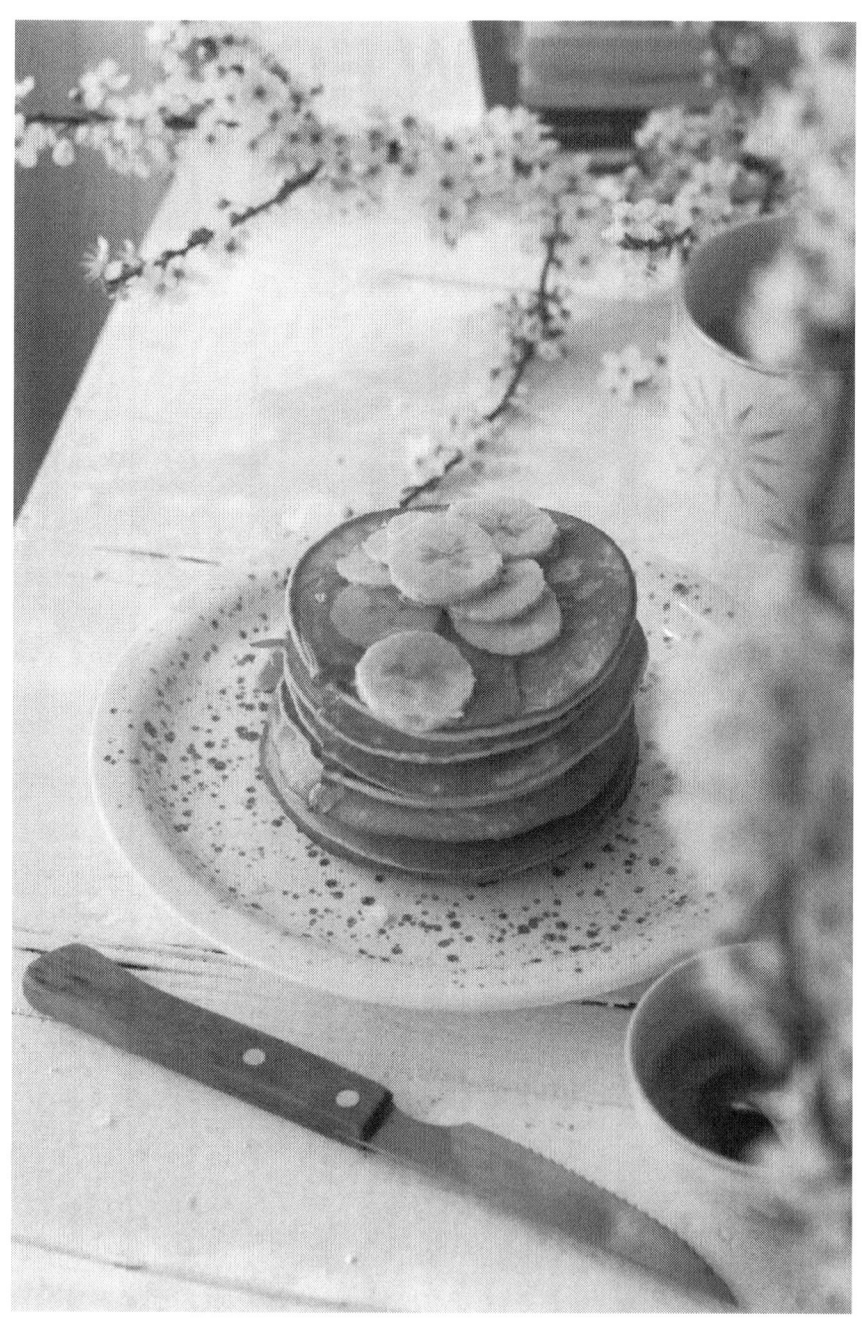

Table of Contents

INTRODUCTION 7
   KEY TO A HEALTHY GUT 10
   LOW FODMAP DIET AS A LIFESTYLE 12
   WHAT CAUSES IBS AND DIGESTIVE DISORDERS 14
   LOW FODMAP DIET TARGETS & BENEFITS 18
   LIST OF INGREDIENTS TO AVOID 20
   BEST TIPS TO SUCCEED IN THE KITCHEN WITH LOW FODMAP DIET 23
   POSITIVE VIBES FROM THE AUTHOR 26

RECIPES 28
   EASY BREAKFAST & SMOOTHIES 29
      Quiche Breakfast Bake 30
      Cornbread Waffles 32
      Salmon Scrambled Eggs 34
      Strawberry & Kiwi Smoothie 36
      Choco Breakfast Bowl 38
      Spinach & Eggs Omelette 40
      Potato & Zucchini Hash Browns 42
      Breakfast Tortilla 44
      Green Detox Smoothie-Juice 46
      Breakfast Stuffed Sweet Potatoes 48
      Almond Meal & Banana Pancakes 50
      Sage Breakfast Sausage 52
      Quinoa Breakfast Jar 54
      Pineapple & Carrot Smoothie 56
      Chocolate & Coffee Smoothie 58
   QUICK SOUPS & SALADS 60
      Easy Spinach Soup 61
      Asian Quinoa Salad 63
      Carrot & Potato Soup 65

Spicy Tomato & Pepper Soup 67
Grilled Chicken & Berry Salad 69
Carrot & Parsnip Soup 71
Pasta & Shrimp Salad 73
Cream of Chicken Soup 75
Spicy Potato & Eggs Salad 77
Beef & Veggie Soup 79
Seared Steak & Pepper Salad 81
Chicken Curry Noodle Soup 83
Feta Cheese & Olives Quinoa Salad 85
Salmon Chowder 87
Nicoise Salad 89

HEALTHY VEGAN & VEGETARIAN MAINS 91
Veggie & Tofu Kebab 92
Veggies Frittata 95
Thai Pumpkin Noodles 97
Sweet Potato Oven Fries & Salad 100
Curry Quinoa Patties 103
Low Fodmap Pizza 106
Egg & Veggie Wraps 108
Egg Shakshuka 110
Basil & Spinach Pesto Risotto 112
Vegan Tofu Masala 114
Veggie "Meatballs" & Salad 116
Fish & Seafood 119
Mediterranean Fish Stew 120
Seafood Risotto 122
Curry Calamari 125
Pepper & Shrimps Pasta 127
Broiled Tilapia Fillets 129
Tuna & Sweet Potato Patties 131
Salmon & Mini Potatoes 133
Tomato Fish Soup 135

Fish Pie 137
Soy Glazed Salmon & Sesame 140
Poultry & Meat.. 142
Chicken Piccata.. 143
Low Fodmap Beef Stew 145
Pesto Chicken Kebabs 147
Pork Chops in Bacon Mustard Sauce & Mashed Potatoes 149
Lamb & Spinach Curry 151
Beef & Broccoli... 153
Chicken & Pork Meatloaf 155
Sausage, Peppers & Eggs 158
Sweet Potato, Chicken & Veggies Bake............. 160
Spicy Lamb Meatballs & Pumpkin Mush 162
Sesame Chicken Bites 165
Stuffed Beef Peppers 168
Pork Stir-Fry & Noodles...................................... 170
Greek-Style Chicken Thighs............................... 172
Italian Meatballs & Zucchini Noodles.................. 174
Easy Turkey Roast 177
Low Fodmap BBQ Pork Chops 179
Chicken Stuffed with Spinach & Ricotta Cheese 181
Pumpkin Beef Chili 184
Peanut Butter Chicken.. 186

SWEET SNACKS & DESSERTS 188
Low FODMAP Carrot Energy Balls..................... 189
Chocolate Brownies.. 191
Low FODMAP Lemon Cake 193
Easy No-Bake Cookies....................................... 196
Low FODMAP Pumpkin Pie Mousse 198
Fruit Salad 200
Stovetop Sweet Popcorn 202
Carrot Cake 204

    Chocolate, Peanut Butter & Roasted Bananas . 206
    Easy Matcha Pudding 208

3-WEEK MEAL PLAN 210

    1ST WEEK: 210
    2ND WEEK: 211
    3RD WEEK: 212

CONCLUSION 213

Introduction

While the vast majority of diets nowadays focus on weight loss rather than health benefits, some new diet types have landed to change the diet realm for good. The low FODMAP diet is a fairly new diet pattern that is gaining popularity because of its special health benefits. The diet was originally mentioned in an Australian diet journal around 2006 and has now achieved global recognition as a dietary option to treat Irritable Bowel Syndrome (IBS) and possibly other digestive disorders. So, what is the Low FODMAP diet about? The name "FODMAP" refers to "Fermentable Oligosaccharides, Disaccharides, Monosaccharides, & Polyols"-these are all types of short-chained carbs that are fermentable and poorly absorbed by the system, often leading to digestive problems. They are partially fermented in the large intestine but are slowly and poorly absorbed by the system. Hence, a low FODMAP diet is a diet choice that limits the consumption of these carbs from certain foods and replaces them with lower FODMAP alternatives (foods that contain lower amounts of these carb types).

FODMAPs in food can occur either naturally or artificially as additives. They contain some types of sugars and alcohols e.g. fructose, lactose (from some dairy), gas (from nuts), fructans (from certain fruits and veggies), and polyols (from natural or artificial sweeteners).

According to official diet guidelines and suggestions, the diet is followed in 3 separate stages which last anywhere from 3-8 weeks max:

- The Elimination Phase. This is the first stage of the diet which typically lasts 2-6 weeks and during this phase, you are allowed to eat foods that are low or very low in FODMAPS. This is the most restrictive phase.
- The Re-Introduction/Sensitivity Phase. At this phase, which lasts 4-8 weeks or doubles the time of the initial phase, foods that are higher in FODMAPS are gradually introduced to determine sensitivities and reactions to certain high FODMAP foods.
- The Personalization Phase. This is the final stage with no particular timeframe where the person has already determined the FODMAP foods that worsen their digestive problems and control their consumption while re-introducing other foods that may be high in FODMAPS to increase tolerance.

As evident from the re-introduction and personalization phase, each person may react differently to certain foods with a high FODMAP content--some for example may find that high-fructose foods agitate their digestive problems while for others lactose and dairy is often the culprit of their systems. Hence, there is no point in eliminating all high-FODMAP foods for long periods as this will be too restrictive and deprive the body of vital nutrients.

In the present eBook, we are going to give you a list of low FODMAP foods so you can consume them in the first elimination stage which will last 3 weeks. Our 3-week meal plan will give you a clear idea of what to eat during this stage so you don't have to figure out which foods and recipes to prepare and eat on your own. After All, we have included 80 delicious low FODMAP recipes to try out so there is plenty of room for experimentation--from hearty meaty breakfasts to vegan sweet snacks, there is something for everyone.

Key to a Healthy Gut

Our Gastrointestinal Gut (GI), bowel, or gut has a pivotal role to play in preserving the health and life of our systems. This is the first organic body system that notes rapid growth during the first 3 years of our lives and continues to develop for the rest of our lives. Its primary role is to digest and break down the food we consume and facilitate nutrient absorption or waste/elimination of unwanted substances whenever necessary. Gut was also surprisingly found to have connections with the brain (the gut-brain axis) and the immune system, indirectly affecting their health.

The human gut reportedly hosts over 100 trillion microorganisms, generally known as 'microbiota' or 'microflora'. These include both beneficial and health-preserving bacteria (probiotics) as well as bad bacteria and parasites that may lead to various health symptoms if their population spans out of control.

Essentially, there are two schools of thought when it comes to improving gut health. The first is to increase or feed the population of beneficial bacteria that resides on the gut and the second is the reduction of bad bacteria or elimination of triggering substances from foods that may aggravate gut health. In many cases, these two approaches are used in tandem for deeper and more long-lasting results. This is essentially the key to optimal gut health in the long run.

The low FODMAP diet works by eliminating certain food triggers and depriving the bacterial population of feeding nutrients that they need to survive. However, since the diet might starve bad as well as good bacteria during the elimination phase, it is always a good idea to supplement your diet with probiotics so you don't lose any beneficial bacteria along the process.

Low Fodmap Diet as a Lifestyle

As specified earlier, the low FODMAP diet is not another diet fab for losing weight and getting shredded. It's a lifestyle choice that will improve gut health temporarily or for longer periods, as long as it is followed wisely and in moderation. Since over 50 million Americans suffer from digestive problems on a chronic basis and the global prevalence according to multinational studies reaches 40% of the adult population, it would be wise to follow a diet and lifestyle that improves chronic gut health.

IBS especially is a common disturbance that affects over 25 million Americans and approx. 15% of the total population worldwide. Common symptoms include bloating, gas, and abdominal pain. The symptoms can range from mild to severe and in some cases they are so extreme that they cause disability and failure to keep up with daily life tasks e.g work. Hence, a diet that manages these symptoms e.g the low FODMAP diet, is a diet that will give the sufferers their normal life back.

Many mistakenly think that the low FODMAP diet is only about the elimination of high FODMAP foods to control IBS symptoms but this isn't the case. The diet is only a part of a more holistic approach to achieving gut health. Paired with a healthy lifestyle e.g no smoking, decreased stress, the effects of the diet will be more profound and lasting.

What Causes IBS and Digestive Disorders

Patients and doctors have noticed for quite a long time that certain foods and substances may trigger IBS and similar digestive symptoms e.g, gas, bloating irregular bowel movements. Some well-known food triggers, as mentioned earlier are lactose, fructose, alcohol, etc. These are often found in certain dairy products, legumes, nuts, grains, cruciferous veggies, and fruits. Some of these have been found to cause gas and should be avoided in cases of vivid bloating and indigestion. However, up until a few decades ago, these certain foods appeared in the lists of foods to avoid for IBS without exactly identifying the common chemical attributes that these food triggers shared. Eventually, with the progress of science and technology that took off the last 40 years, these chemical substances were identified and classified as potential triggers for people who experience IBS and other digestive problems. The poor digestion and malabsorption of these short-chain carbs have been described by medical researchers as the culprit of gas, bloating, diarrhea, nausea, and abdominal pain in patients diagnosed with IBS. The earliest reports have identified 5 particular culprits, categorized based on their chemical form:

- **Lactose.** Early studies that date back to the 50s and 60s have found a link between lactose and diarrhea symptoms. Ever since there have been numerous lab diagnostic means to check lactose responses and diagnose intolerance. In intolerant patients with digestive issues, doctors have advised the elimination of lactose from the patient's diet, however, this has been found to ease only some symptoms of IBS and not solve the matter completely.
- **Fructose & Sorbitol.** Fructose is a type of monosaccharide sugar that is naturally found in fruits. Sorbitol is also similar to sugar alcohol and carb found in certain fruits like figs and plums. Although not many studies have found a clear link between fructose/sorbitol and IBS symptoms, a few studies have found that fructose or low fructose and sorbitol diet has eased IBS symptoms in patients that didn't respond to other methods of treatment or lactose elimination.
- **Oligosaccharides.** Oligosaccharides (oligos or oligo-fructans) stand for the "O" in "FODMAP" and refer to sugar alcohols that contain up to 10

linked monosaccharide units--in simple words, they are classified as "simple sugars". These include both natural and artificial sweeteners. Beans and some veggies e.g Jerusalem artichokes are also high in oligos. Our systems though have been found to lack the enzymes necessary to digest and fully absorb oligos, resulting in flatulence (gas) and constipation.

- **Polyols.** Polyols (standing for the "P" in FODMAP) are sugar alcohols that occur naturally in certain fruits and artificial sweeteners like mannitol and xylitol. Their ability to aggravate gut symptoms was first discovered in a 60s study and there have been studies ever since backing up the link between polyps and induced gut symptoms, especially when combined with fructose and sorbitol. However, in moderate doses polyps have been found to have a beneficial effect on the gut's biome, increasing the numbers of beneficial bacteria in the gut.

The common pattern here is that these substances lead collectively to indigestion (lactose), malabsorption (fructose, sorbitol, polyols), and fermentation (oligos) which ultimately lead to IBS and digestive disorders when they are consumed in high amounts.

Stress and other lifestyle factors may also be clear culprits of IBS symptoms; however, a few studies have found that they may worsen already existing symptoms in IBS-affected patients.

Therefore, a low FODMAP diet followed periodically coupled with a healthy lifestyle may be the answer for the effective reduction of IBS symptoms.

Low Fodmap Diet Targets & Benefits

By now, you already realize that the main purpose of a low FODMAP diet is to treat IBS and other digestive problems. A short-term or occasionally followed low FODMAP diet has been found to effectively treat the symptoms that come with the fermentation, indigestion, or malabsorption of certain carbs and substances in those who are intolerant to these. More specifically, a low FODMAP diet can result in:

- Less gas/flatulence. Due to the decreased fermentation of sugar carbs in the digestive tract, the system will be able to release less gas. In one particular UK study, it has been found that 87% of the study participants who followed a low FODMAP diet have noted a significant decrease in gas production/flatulence as opposed to 49% of the control group.
- Less bloating. In the same study above, the study's subjects who followed a low FODMAP diet have shown an impressive decrease of their bloating symptoms by as much as 82% compared

to 49% of those that did not follow the low FODMAP diet.
- Less abdominal pain. In a study involving big children aged 7-18, it has been found that the children who followed a low FODMAP diet had less intense abdominal pain episodes compared to the children participants who followed another diet type (TACD).
- Less diarrhea. A US study conducted in 110 adult patients with diarrhea-predominant IBS symptoms, has shown that the patients' group who followed a low FODMAP diet had fewer diarrhea episodes and noted better stool frequency than those who followed a GDA (Guideline Daily Amounts) diet.

Although symptoms and their severity may vary between IBS patients, there is plenty of evidence pointing out significant improvements in bloating, gas, abdominal pain, and diarrhea in patients who follow the diet for a few weeks. Therefore, if you experience any of the above, your symptoms will most likely improve, if you follow the low FODMAP diet properly.

List of Ingredients to Avoid

The actual foods and ingredients that are high on FODMAPS and may, in turn, aggravate IBS symptoms are the following (we have broken this down to 5 main categories and subcategories so you can check easily which foods to avoid when you are in the first stage of the low FODMAP diet).

Fruits:
- Apples
- Apricots
- Blackberries
- Cherries
- Mangoes
- Nectarines
- Pears
- Plums
- Prunes
- Watermelon
- Dried fruits e.g. apricots, figs, etc.

Vegetables:
- Artichokes
- Asparagus
- Beetroot

- Broccoli
- Brussel sprouts
- Cauliflower
- Celery
- Garlic
- Leeks
- Mushrooms
- Onions
- Sweet Corn

Legumes:
- Beans (all kinds)
- Lentils

Nuts:
- Cashew Nuts
- Pistachios

Sugars:
- Agave nectar
- Corn Syrup
- Fructose
- Honey
- Maltitol
- Sorbitol
- Xylitol

Wheat products (with gluten):
- Cereals
- Crackers
- Bread
- Pasta
- Pizza

Dairy:
- Cow milk
- Custard
- Ice cream
- Pudding
- Soft cheeses e.g cottage cheese
- Yogurt

Drinks:
- Alcohol
- Sports & energy drinks with artificial sweeteners

Best Tips to Succeed In the Kitchen With Low Fodmap Diet

Following a low FODMAP diet can be a tad challenging for newbies; however, don't let the list of "foods to avoid" fool you and limit your cooking options. There are just as many if not more cooking ingredients to explore and you can prepare low FODMAP meals much easier if you follow these kitchen tips. Here they are:

Tip #1: Prepare your meals in advance. If you don't have the time and energy to prepare your low FODMAP meal for the day, choose 1-2 days a week based on your schedule to prepare a week's worth of low FODMAP meals in advance. Make a shopping list of what you'll need (in case you don't have the necessary recipe ingredients already), go shopping, and spare 2-3 hours every time to prepare your weekly meals. You can also keep any leftovers in the freezer if you plan to prepare larger batches of food.

Tip#2: Make your condiments and dressings. Most store-bought condiments and dressings e.g ketchup contain hidden amounts of processed or natural sugars which are the worst triggering FODMAPs for IBS patients. If you are not sure whether a condiment or dressing is low FODMAP, check its label and avoid anything that contains corn syrup, maltitol, fructose, or any other sugar from the prohibited list. If the recipe calls it, prepare your own using natural ingredients and low FODMAP sweetener alternatives such as maple syrup or Stevia.

Tip#3: Go for lactose-free dairy options. There is no need to quit eating dairy altogether when you are on a low FODMAP diet as there are some dairy options that contain low to zero amounts of lactose and thus are low on FODMAPs. Some good low or lactose-free options include dry/mature cheeses, lactose-free milk, and lactose-free yogurt. Vegetarian dairy alternatives like almond milk and soy yogurt are perfectly fine as long as they don't contain any FODMAP sugar types.

Tip#4: Use spices in place of onions and garlic. Avoiding onions and garlic is a bit challenging as most recipes nowadays use these to add some flavor and dimension to the dish, however, you can counteract their lack by using flavorful spices e.g. curry, coriander, cumin, chili flakes. Nearly all spices (apart from garlic and onion powder obviously) are perfectly fine to use in a low FODMAP diet and there is no limit to their amounts--it's a matter of how hot or spicy you like your food.

Tip#5: Saute your meat and veggies first. In addition to using spices in your dishes in place of onion and garlic, you can add more flavor to your dishes by browning your meat and veggies first in a bit of vegetable oil. You can also make your onion and garlic-free stock by browning low FODMAP veggies e.g carrots and parsnips and adding at least 4 cups of boiling water, salt, herbs, and spices. Once your stock is ready, you can keep it in the fridge for up to 1 week (to use later on your weekly meals) or in the freezer for up to 2 months, in the form of ice-cubes so you can use 1-2 cubes every time you need it for the recipe.

Positive Vibes from the Author

Following a low FODMAP diet isn't as challenging as some people assume. If you prepare your meals in advance, check your portions, and experiment with low FODMAP alternatives for at least a week, things will be much easier afterward. Keep in mind that during the final stages, you may re-introduce some foods that are higher in FODMAPs to see your gut's reaction, and based on our research, most people are affected by one type of FODMAP more than others. So don't worry, you won't have to quit eating all the foods on the prohibited list for long periods and restrict yourself.

And if you are stuck or don't know what else you should cook, check out our recipes or join an online FODMAP diet community to draw some inspiration and support from people like you who are already following the diet. Even better, you may seek the professional advice and support of a nutritionist who has experience in treating patients with digestive disorders, especially IBS. Don't be afraid to ask for help; sometimes it's best to have someone on your side instead of going through your diet journey alone.

Remember: Low FODMAP is not just another diet fad, it's a lifestyle choice and your gut will thank you for it!

Recipes

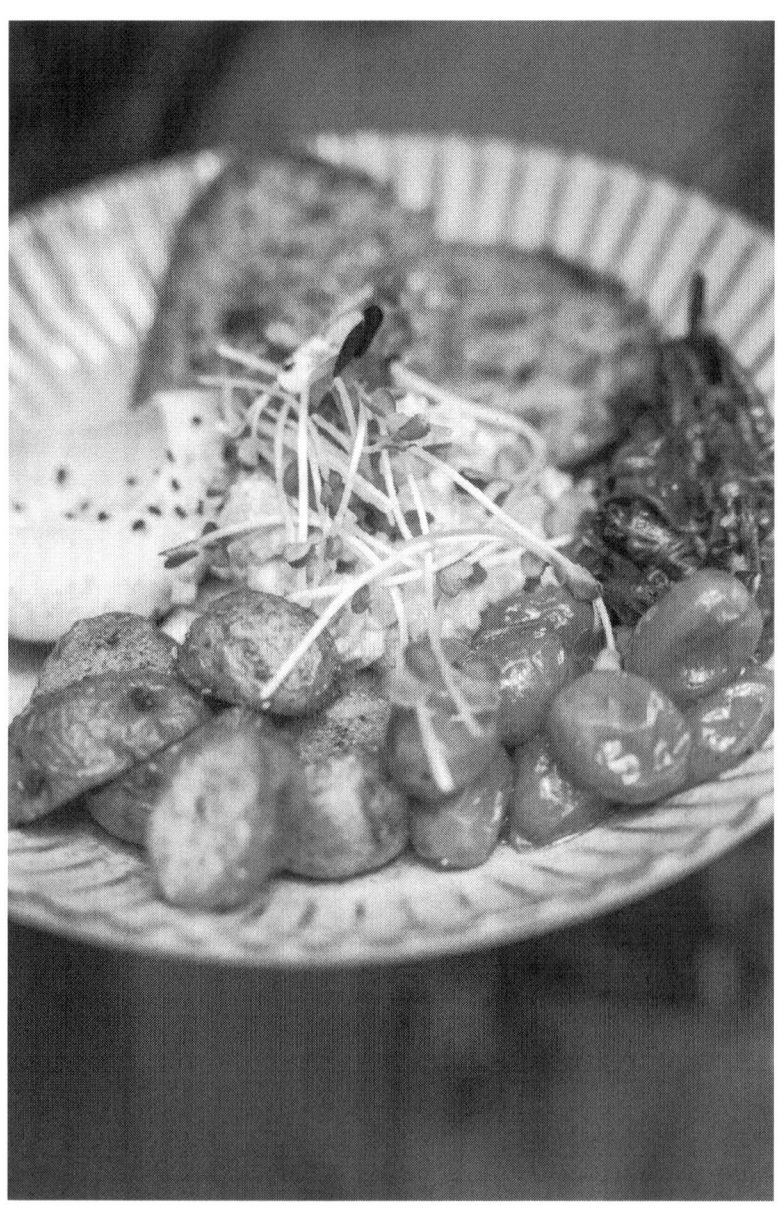

Easy Breakfast & Smoothies

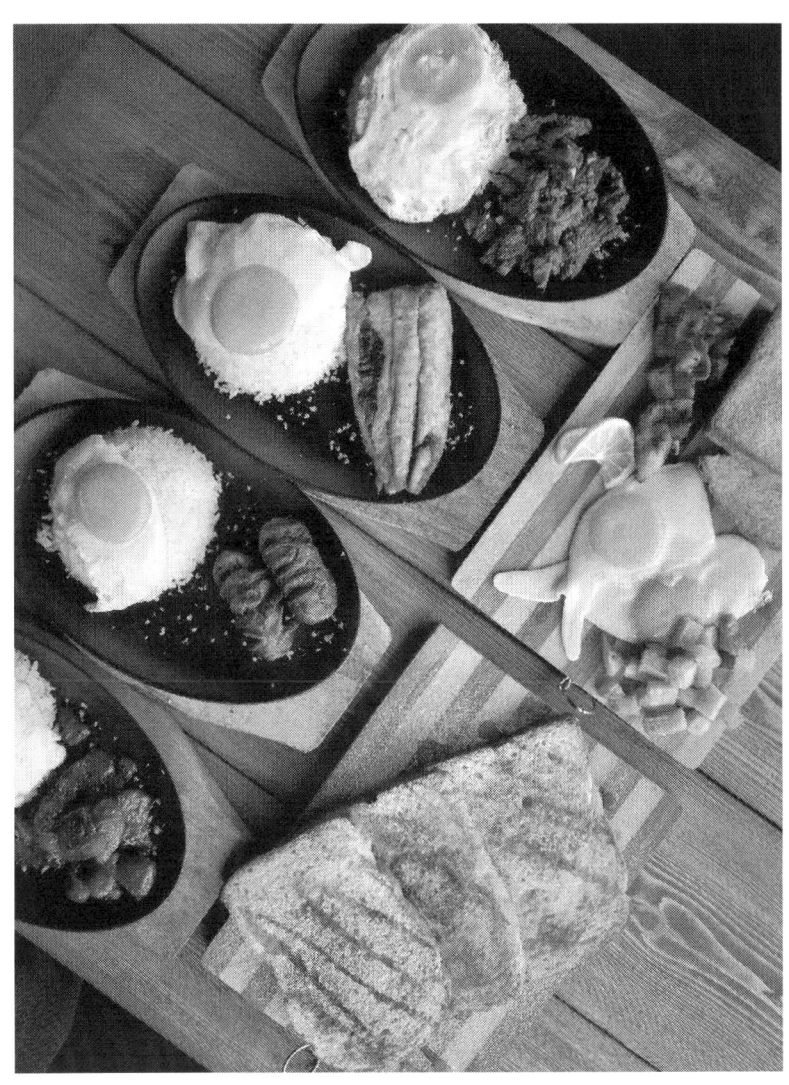

Quiche Breakfast Bake

A hearty breakfast bake that resembles the flavors and texture of quiche, minus the crust. A great breakfast or brunch that will fill you up for hours.

Cuisine: American

Ingredients for 6 Servings

- 10 whole eggs, beaten
- 1 cup (240ml) soy or veggie cream
- 1 cup (30g) fresh spinach leaves
- 6 cherry tomatoes, halved
- 1 tsp chili flakes
- ½ cup (117g) mature cheddar cheese, shredded
- 1 tsp mustard powder
- Salt and pepper
- Olive oil

Cooking Time: 30 min

Directions

1. Beat the eggs with the soy or veggie cream well and add the spices. Season with salt and pepper.
2. Grease the bottom of a 7X11" or 8X8" baking dish with olive oil. Preheat your oven to 390F/199C for 5 minutes.
3. Combine the egg mixture with spinach and

tomatoes and top with the cheddar cheese.
4. Bake at 400F/204C for approx. 30 minutes.

Nutritional Info (Per Serving)

Calories: 232kcal

Total Fat: 16.6g

Saturated Fat:5.2g

Cholesterol: 282mg

Carbs: 7g

Protein: 12.3g

Sodium: 247mg

Fiber: 0.6g

Vitamins

A, K, C

Cornbread Waffles

A gluten and lactose-free version of the famous Southern cornbread waffles with almond milk, cornmeal, and oat flour.

Cuisine: Belgian-American

Ingredients for 2 Servings (2 large waffles)

- ½ cup (70g) cornmeal
- ½ cup (70g) oat or fine almond flour
- ¾ cup (180ml) unsweetened almond milk
- 1 large egg, beaten
- 1 tsp baking powder
- 2 tbsp butter, melted
- 1 drizzle of maple syrup
- Greasing spray
- Strawberries (for serving)

Cooking Time: 15 min

Directions

1. Preheat your waffle maker or pan and grease with cooking spray.
2. Mix all the dry ingredients in a bowl (flours, powder).
3. In a separate bowl, beat the eggs with the almond milk and the melted butter. Incorporate with the

dry ingredient mixture and stir well.
4. Let the waffle batter sit for 7-8 minutes at room temperature or until it rises in volume and becomes a bit bubbly.
5. Make sure your waffle maker or waffle pan is hot enough and greased properly. Pour half of the batter with a scoop into your waffle maker/pan and spread evenly with a spatula.
6. Press and let cook over medium heat until golden brown and crisp on the outside (around 2 minutes).
7. Let cool and serve with a drizzle of maple syrup and some strawberries on top.

Nutritional Info (Per Serving)

Calories: 466 kcal

Total Fat:18.3g

Saturated Fat:8.5g

Cholesterol:124mg

Carbs: 65.3g

Protein: 10.4g

Sodium: 202mg

Fiber:3.8g

Vitamins

B-12, B2, C

Salmon Scrambled Eggs

An easy yet incredibly delicious version of scrambled eggs with salmon, dill, and capers.

Cuisine: American

Ingredients for 2 Servings

- 4 large whole eggs
- 1 slice (20-25g) smoked salmon, cut into strips
- 1 tbsp capers
- ½ tsp fresh or dried dill
- 1 tbsp soy cream
- ½ tsp lemon zest
- 1 tbsp vegetable oil
- Salt and pepper

Cooking Time: 5 min

Directions

1. Beat the eggs with soy cream and add salt and pepper.
2. Heat the oil in a shallow pan over low to medium heat and add the eggs. Begin to stir with a spatula to scramble the eggs.
3. Once the eggs are nearly set (with a bit of moisture left) stir in the smoked salmon, the capers, and dill. Continue to cook for about half a

minute.
4. Serve with a bit of lemon zest on top.

Nutritional Info (Per Serving)

Calories: 225kcal

Total Fat: 16.9g

Saturated Fat: 4.3g

Cholesterol: 374mg

Carbs: 2.4g

Protein: 15.3g

Sodium: 566mg

Fiber: 0.6g

Vitamins

B2, B12, A, K

Strawberry & Kiwi Smoothie

A zesty smoothie for those who want to kick start their day with something sweet and sour, minus the guilt. A perfect smoothie for summer mornings.

Cuisine: International

Ingredients for 2 Servings (2 jars)
- 1 ripe kiwi, peeled
- 4 large strawberries, halved
- 1 cup (250ml) unsweetened almond milk
- ½ cup (125ml) water
- 1 tsp maple syrup
- ½ tsp vanilla powder
- 4 ice cubes

Cooking Time: 2 min

Directions
1. Blend everything in a blender or smoothie maker until nice and smooth.
2. Serve chilled into 2 medium-size glasses or mason jars.

Nutritional Info (Per Serving, 1 jar)

Calories: 110kcal

Total Fat: 4.2g

Saturated Fat: 2.2g

Cholesterol: 12mg

Carbs: 13.1g

Protein: 4.6g

Sodium: 57mg

Fiber: 1.4g

Vitamins

C,B2,B12

Choco Breakfast Bowl

A healthy and satisfying breakfast bowl recipe with chocolate chips, peanut butter, banana soaked in oats overnight.

Cuisine: International

Ingredients for 1 Serving

- 2 tbsp rolled oats
- ½ cup (123ml) oat or almond milk
- 1 tbsp unsweetened peanut butter
- 1 tbsp chocolate chips
- 1 small semi-ripe banana, sliced

Cooking Time: Overnight

Directions

1. Mix the rolled oats with the oat or almond milk in a bowl or large mason jar. Make sure that all oats are saturated with the mixture, using a small spoon or spatula.
2. Top the mixture with peanut butter, chocolate chips, and finally banana slices.
3. Leave the mixture on your fridge overnight or for at least 3 hours. Serve chilled.

Nutritional Info (Per Serving)

Calories: 351kca

Total Fat: 10.3g

Saturated Fat: 1.5g

Cholesterol: 0mg

Carbs: 65.9g

Protein: 5.5g

Sodium: 355mg

Fiber: 5.6g

Vitamins

B12, E, C

Spinach & Eggs Omelette

An easy and delicious omelette with good-for-you spinach and few "secret" ingredients that amplify its taste without being noticeable.

Cuisine: International

Ingredients for 2 Servings
- 5 medium eggs, beaten
- 1 cup (30g) spinach leaves
- 1 tsp tomato paste
- ½ tsp lemon pepper
- Salt and Pepper
- 2 tbsp olive oil
- A drizzle of hot sauce

Cooking Time: 7-8 min

Directions
1. Beat the eggs with the tomato paste well (preferably in a blender or food processor).
2. Heat the olive oil in a medium pan and add the spinach. Season with lemon pepper, salt, and pepper to taste. Cook until wilted (around 2 minutes). Take off the heat and strain from all the liquids.
3. Add the spinach back to the pan and add the

eggs. Spread everything evenly with a spatula. Cook the omelette until eggs are set on both sides or until you achieve a golden-brown crust.
4. Cut the omelette in half and serve with a drizzle of hot sauce on top.

Nutritional Info (Per Serving)

Calories: 293kcal

Total Fat: 24.1g

Saturated Fat:5.3g

Cholesterol: 409mg

Carbs: 4.1g

Protein: 14.7g

Sodium: 447mg

Fiber: 0.9g

Vitamins

A, K, C

Potato & Zucchini Hash Browns

A delicious hash brown recipe with shredded potato and zucchini, with the right amount of crunch.

Cuisine: American

Ingredients for 6 small patties
- 1 large russet potato, peeled and shredded
- 1 small zucchini, shredded
- 1 tsp thyme
- 1 small egg
- 1 tbsp corn-starch
- Salt and pepper
- 3 tbsp vegetable oil

Cooking Time: 8 min

Directions
1. Squeeze the shredded potato and zucchini with your hands to remove any liquids and transfer to a dish with kitchen paper to absorb excess moisture.
2. Combine the potato, zucchini, egg, and corn-starch in a bowl. Season with thyme, salt, and pepper.

3. Heat the oil in a pan. Take a large spoon and form the mixture into 5-6 equal-size patties. Transfer the patties with a spatula into the pan.
4. Cook the patties for approx. 2 minutes on each side or until golden brown. Cook in 2 batches of 3 patties each.

Nutritional Info (Per Serving, 1 pattie)

Calories: 128kcal

Total Fat: 7.5g

Saturated Fat: 1.2g

Cholesterol: 24mg

Carbs: 13.2g

Protein: 2.4g

Sodium: 429mg

Fiber: 1.1g

Vitamins

C, B6, A

Breakfast Tortilla

A hearty breakfast tortilla wraps with eggs, sausage, and 2 pepper kinds, with a touch of Tex-Mex seasonings.

Cuisine: Tex-Mex

Ingredients for 2 tortilla wraps

- 2 medium-size corn tortillas
- 6 eggs, beaten
- 1 slice spicy sausage, sliced
- 1 small red bell pepper, sliced
- ½ small green bell pepper, sliced
- ½ tsp cumin
- ½ tsp paprika
- 1 tsp hot sauce
- 2 tbsp vegetable oil
- Salt and pepper

Cooking Time: 8 min

Directions

1. Heat the oil in a medium pan and add the sliced peppers. Saute until slightly softened (but still a bit crunchy) for around 2 minutes.
2. Add the sausage and saute for another minute or so.

3. Add the eggs and the spices and season with salt and pepper. Stir and scramble everything with a spatula. Cook until the eggs are set.
4. Distribute the egg mixture into 2 warm tortillas, add the hot sauce, and wrap folding the edges inwards (as if you are making a packet or burrito). Serve hot.

Nutritional Info (Per Serving, 1 tortilla)

Calories: 418kcal

Total Fat: 29.7g

Saturated Fat: 6.8g

Cholesterol: 491mg

Carbs: 17.1g

Protein: 21.3g

Sodium: 345mg

Fiber: 3.2g

Vitamins

A, C, B2

Green Detox Smoothie-Juice

A zesty totally healthy and detoxing smoothie with super-greens, lemon, and kiwi. A sure way to start your day with plenty of energy.

Cuisine: International

Ingredients for 2 Glasses

- ½ cup (20g) spinach leaves
- ½ cup (20g) kale, chopped
- 1 ripe kiwi, peeled
- 1 cup (240ml) unsweetened almond milk
- ½ cup (120ml) chilled water
- 1 tsp maple syrup

Cooking Time: 2 min

Directions

1. Blend all the ingredients until nice and smooth (you will end up with a bright green liquid).
2. Serve chilled into 2 mason jars or glasses.

Nutritional Info (Per Serving, 1 jar)

Calories: 108kcal

Total Fat: 1.5g

Saturated Fat: 0g

Cholesterol: 0mg

Carbs: 23.1

Protein: 1.4g

Sodium: 120mg

Fiber: 0.8g

Vitamins

A, K, B12

Breakfast Stuffed Sweet Potatoes

A quick and easy recipe that combines ideally the sweet and filling flavor of sweet potatoes with eggs and a bit of bacon. Ready in the microwave in under 10 minutes.

Cuisine: American

Ingredients for 2 Servings
- 2 medium sweet potatoes, washed
- 2 eggs
- 1 thick slice of bacon, finely chopped
- 2 tsp butter
- Dash of cinnamon
- Salt and pepper

Cooking Time: 8 min

Directions
1. Slash the upper surface of the sweet potato with a small knife, making a cross-section. Pinch with a fork, making small holes everywhere.
2. Pop in the microwave for 6 minutes (medium to high heat).
3. Once the core of the sweet potatoes is soft,

spoon out some flesh to transfer the eggs (crack one egg into each potato). Add the butter, cinnamon, salt, and pepper, and top with the bacon bits.
4. Cook in the microwave for another 2-3 minutes or until eggs are set. Serve hot.

Nutritional Info (Per Serving)

Calories: 277kcal

Total Fat: 13.4g

Saturated Fat:3.8g

Cholesterol:174mg

Carbs: 30.4g

Protein:9.6g

Sodium: 282mg

Fiber:4.9g

Vitamins

A, C, B5

Almond Meal & Banana Pancakes

A simple and healthy variation of pancakes, with almond meal and banana to add a bit of low FODMAP sweetness.

Cuisine: American

Ingredients for 4 Servings
- 1 ½ cup (218g) blanched almond flour
- 2 semi-ripe bananas, mashed with a fork
- 4 large eggs, yolks, and whites separated
- ½ tsp baking powder
- Greasing spray
- Maple syrup

Cooking Time: 15 min

Directions
1. Take two mixing bowls and keep the egg yolks and whites separately. Beat the egg whites well with a whisk or a hand mixer until white and fluffy.
2. In the second bowl, beat the egg yolks with the bananas and baking powder. Once mixed well, gently fold in the foamy egg whites with a spatula (do not over mix) into the egg yolk mixture.

3. Add almond flour, mix gently.
4. Grease the bottom of a small pan with greasing spray. Add ¼ of the mixture each time, flatten out with a spatula and cook the pancake until golden brown on both sides. Repeat the above step (making sure to grease the pan every time) until you finish all the batter.
5. Serve your pancakes with a drizzle of maple syrup on top.

Nutritional Info (Per Serving)

Calories: 457kcal

Total Fat: 36.1g

Saturated Fat:4.1g

Cholesterol:184mg

Carbs: 25.3g

Protein: 14.8g

Sodium:20mg

Fiber: 6.6g

Vitamins

E, B2, B6

Sage Breakfast Sausage

A delicious savory breakfast recipe with ground pork, sage, parsley, and a hint of mustard.

Cuisine: American

Ingredients for 4 patties
- 1 lb. (450g) ground pork
- 1 tsp sage
- ½ tsp thyme
- 1 tbsp mustard
- 1 tbsp lemon juice
- Salt and pepper
- 3 tbsp vegetable oil

Cooking Time: 7-8 min

Directions
1. Combine the ground pork with sage, thyme, lemon juice, mustard, and salt/pepper. Shape into 4 medium round patties.
2. Heat the vegetable oil in a pan. Once the oil gets hot, add the patties. Cook for approx. 3 minutes on each side and serve.

Nutritional Info (Per Serving)
Calories: 290kcal

Total Fat: 22.6g

Saturated Fat: 6.9g

Cholesterol: 91mg

Carbs: 1.1g

Protein: 19.6g

Sodium: 500mg

Fiber:0.3g

Vitamins

B1, B6, C

Quinoa Breakfast Jar

A super nutritious and deliciously sweet breakfast in a jar with tri-color quinoa, strawberries, and chocolate shavings.

Cuisine: International

Ingredients for 1 Serving

- ½ cup (90g) tri-color quinoa
- 1 cup water
- ¼ cup (60ml) almond milk
- 4 strawberries, halved
- 1 tsp maple syrup
- 1 tbsp chocolate shavings

Cooking Time: 20 min

Directions

1. Wash and rinse the quinoa well before cooking.
2. Cook in plain boiling water for 15 minutes, over medium heat.
3. Let the quinoa cool down to room temperature. Add the almond milk, stir, and top with the strawberries and chocolate shavings.
4. Serve with maple syrup.

Nutritional Info (Per Serving)

Calories: 555kcal

Total Fat: 18.8g

Saturated Fat: 7.9g

Cholesterol: 1mg

Carbs: 82,1g

Protein: 15.4g

Sodium: 59mg

Fiber: 10.4g

Vitamins

B6, C, B12

Pineapple & Carrot Smoothie

A zesty exotic smoothie with a vibrant orange hue, packed with vitamins and digestive enzymes.

Cuisine: International

Ingredients for 2 Servings

- 2 round slices of fresh pineapple
- 1 small carrot, shredded
- 1 ½ cup (368ml) almond milk
- ½ cup (120ml) chilled water
- 1 tsp stevia

Cooking Time: 2 min

Directions

1. Combine all the ingredients in a blender. Pulse until creamy and smooth.
2. Serve chilled into 2 medium glasses or mason jars.

Nutritional Info (Per Serving)

Calories: 128kcal

Total Fat: 2.3g

Saturated Fat: 0g

Cholesterol: 0mg

Carbs: 31.6g

Protein: 1.5g

Sodium: 147mg

Fiber: 1.8g

Vitamins

A, B12, B2

Chocolate & Coffee Smoothie

A delicious smoothie recipe that incorporates the rich and awakening flavors and aroma of coffee with the chocolate. A perfect way to start your day with the right dose of caffeine.

Cuisine: International

Ingredients for 2 glasses

- 1 cup (240ml) prepared filter coffee or 1.5 shots of espresso diluted in 1 ½ cup of water
- 1 tsp cocoa powder, diluted in 1 tbsp hot water
- 1 semi-ripe banana
- ½ tsp vanilla extract
- ½ cup (123ml) chilled almond milk
- 8 ice-cubes

Cooking Time: 5 min

Directions

1. Make sure the coffee is cool or at room temperature.
2. Blend the coffee, cocoa, banana, almond milk, and vanilla extract in a blender until smooth and creamy.
3. Add the ice-cubes and serve into 2 medium glasses or jars with 4 ice-cubes in each.

Nutritional Info (Per Serving)

Calories: 95kcal

Total Fat: 1.62g

Saturated Fat:0.4g

Cholesterol:0g

Carbs: 18.2g

Protein: 2.7g

Sodium: 49mg

Fiber: 2.1g

Vitamins

B-complex, A, C

Quick Soups & Salads

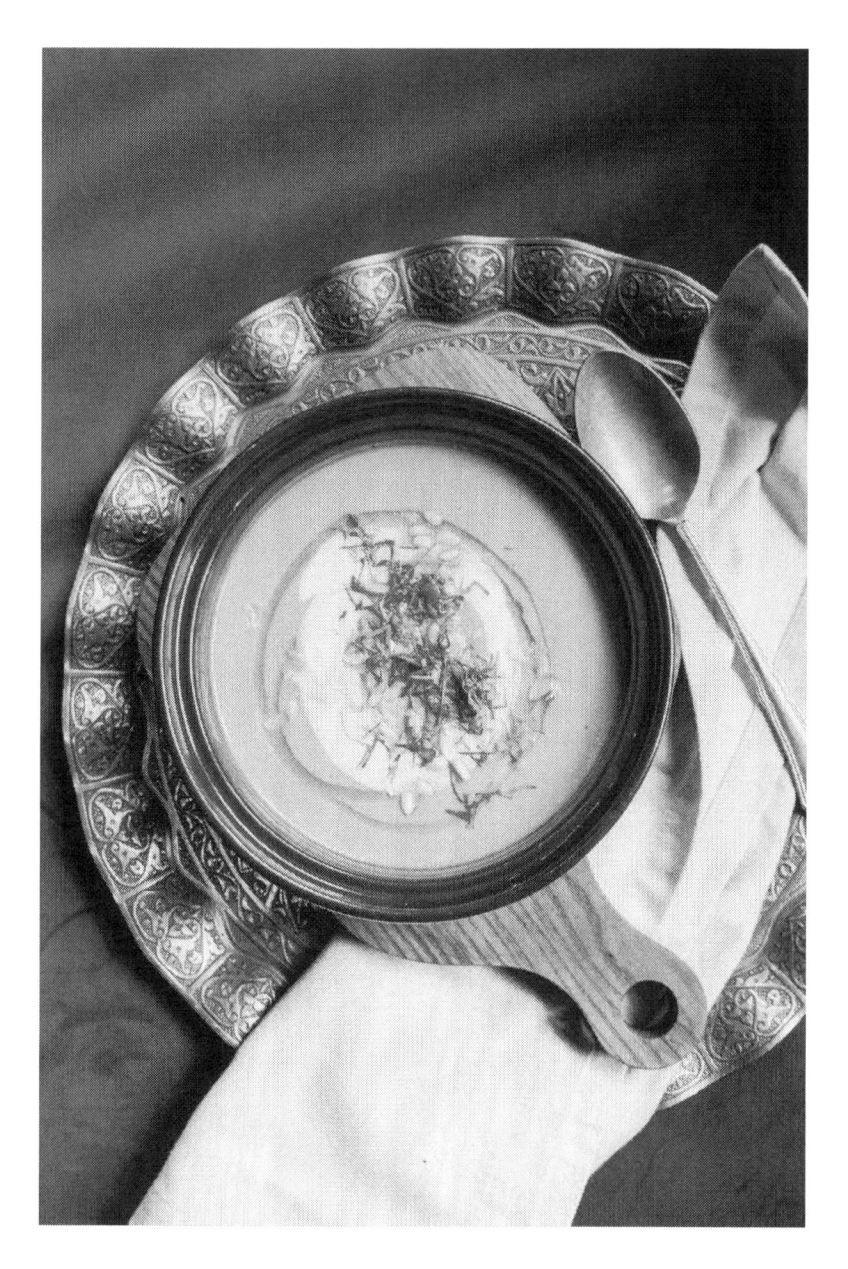

Easy Spinach Soup

An incredibly easy and fast spinach soup with just 4 ingredients, plus it's vegan but you can optionally add some bacon bits if you are a non-vegan eater.

Cuisine: International

Ingredients for 4 Servings
- 2 cups (80g) spinach leaves
- 4 cups (946ml) vegetable stock
- ½ cup (120ml) soy cream
- 1 tbsp fresh dill, chopped
- Salt and Pepper

Cooking Time: 12 min

Directions
1. Bring the vegetable stock to a boil and add the spinach. Cook for 5 minutes or until spinach is totally soft.
2. Add the soy cream, season with salt and pepper, and blend using an immersion blender.
3. Serve in individual bowls with some dill on top.

Nutritional Info (Per Serving)
Calories: 66kcal
Total Fat: 3.3g

Saturated Fat: 0.6g

Cholesterol: 0mg

Carbs: 8.9g

Protein: 1.1g

Sodium: 1016mg

Fiber: 0.9g

Vitamins

A, C, K

Asian Quinoa Salad

A delicious quinoa salad with an Asian twist that includes peppers, soy sauce, and Chinese spices.

Cuisine: Asian

Ingredients for 2 Servings

- 1 cup (180g) white quinoa, washed and rinsed
- 2 cups (475ml) vegetable stock
- 1 red bell pepper, sliced
- ½ yellow bell pepper, sliced
- 1 tbsp soy sauce
- 1 tbsp rice vinegar
- 1 tsp Chinese spice mix
- Coriander leaves (optional)
- Soybean oil

Cooking Time: 25 min

Directions

1. Bring the vegetable stock to a boil and add the quinoa. Cook for around 15 minutes or until quinoa is cooked and has absorbed all the liquids.
2. Meanwhile, roast the sliced peppers with a bit of soybean oil in your oven's broiler (450F/230C) for 10-12 minutes.

3. Once the quinoa is cooked, mix in the roasted peppers, the soy sauce, the rice vinegar, and Chinese spice mix with a spoon or spatula.
4. Serve with some coriander leaves optionally on top.

Nutritional Info (Per Serving)

Calories: 381kcal

Total Fat: 6.8g

Saturated Fat: 0.8g

Cholesterol: 0mg

Carbs: 66.3g

Protein: 13.6g

Sodium: 1069mg

Fiber: 7.8g

Vitamins

A, C, B6

Carrot & Potato Soup

A creamy and hearty carrot and potato soup with the right amount of starch and herbs to add a delicate flavor and aroma.

Cuisine: American/French

Ingredients for 4 Servings
- 2 large Yukon gold potatoes, peeled and cubed
- 2 large carrots, peeled and cubed
- 5 cups (1182ml) vegetable stock
- ½ cup (120ml) soy or almond cream
- 1 tsp thyme
- 2 tbsp olive oil
- 1 tbsp pumpkin seeds

Cooking Time: 40 min

Directions
1. Saute the carrot and potato cubes in olive oil in a medium pot for 2-3 minutes.
2. Add the vegetable stock and bring everything to a boil. Let cook for 30-35 minutes or until potatoes and carrots are totally soft and blendable.
3. Add the soy or almond cream and blend everything with an immersion blender (or food processor) until creamy and smooth.

4. Serve with thyme and pumpkin seeds on top.

Nutritional Info (Per Serving)

Calories: 260kcal

Total Fat: 8.1g

Saturated Fat: 1.1g

Cholesterol: 5.4mg

Carbs: 41.5g

Protein: 7.5g

Sodium: 1361kcal

Fiber: 5.4g,

Vitamins

A, C, B6

Spicy Tomato & Pepper Soup

A delicious red soup for fiery and spicy tastes lovers, made with roasted bell peppers and tomatoes.

Cuisine: American

Ingredients for 4 Servings

- 3 large tomatoes, peeled and halved
- 2 red bell peppers, seeded and halved
- 5 cups (1182ml) vegetable broth
- 2 tbsp soy cream
- 1 tsp chili flakes
- 1 tbsp tahini paste
- A drizzle of olive oil
- Salt and pepper

Cooking Time: 35 min

Directions

1. Drizzle the pepper halves with olive oil, season with salt and pepper, and roast in your oven's broiler (450F/230C) for 10-12 minutes.
2. Meanwhile, bring the vegetable stock to a boil in a medium pot over medium heat. Once the peppers are cooked, add the tomatoes and peppers. Let cook for approx. 20 minutes over medium to low heat.

3. Add the soy cream, tahini paste, and chili flakes towards the last 2 minutes of cooking.
4. Blend everything using an immersion blender or transfer it into a food processor. Blend until creamy and smooth with no visible pepper or tomato bits and serve hot.

Nutritional Info (Per Serving)

Calories: 105kcal

Total Fat: 5.6

Saturated Fat: 0.7g

Cholesterol: 0mg

Carbs: 12.7g

Protein: 3.1g

Sodium: 1462mg

Fiber: 2.6g,

Vitamins

C, A, B6

Grilled Chicken & Berry Salad

A satisfying salad with a lettuce/kale base, grilled chicken, and berries for a tart and fresh note.

Cuisine: International

Ingredients for 4 Servings

- 1 large head of lettuce, washed and roughly chopped
- 2 skinless and boneless chicken breasts (divided into 2 pieces each)
- ½ cup (95g) blueberries
- ½ cup (95g) raspberries
- 6 almonds, roughly chopped
- Salt and pepper

Dressing

- 1 tbsp dijon mustard
- 1 tbsp soy sauce
- 3 tbsp olive oil
- 1 tsp maple syrup

Cooking Time: 15 min

Directions

1. Season the chicken breasts with salt and pepper and grill in a grilling pan or oven grill until fully

cooked (but not too dry), for approx. 3-4 minutes on each side.
2. Mix all the dressing ingredients in a small bowl.
3. Assemble your salad by layering the lettuce leaves first, the berries, the dressing, and the chopped almonds.
4. Toss lightly and add the chicken breasts on top before serving.

Nutritional Info (Per Serving)

Calories: 322kcal

Total Fat: 15.4g

Saturated Fat: 2.3g

Cholesterol: 86mg

Carbs: 17.2g

Protein: 29.4g

Sodium: 758mg

Fiber: 4.2g

Vitamins

K, B6, B3

Carrot & Parsnip Soup

A delicious soup made with roasted carrots, orange bell peppers, and parsnips with a hint of herbs to bring out their natural flavors.

Cuisine: American

Ingredients for 4 Servings

- 4 large carrots, peeled and diced
- 2 large parsnips, peeled and thickly sliced
- 2 orange or yellow bell peppers, seeded and halved
- 5 cups (1182ml) vegetable stock
- 1 cup (240ml) soy cream
- 3 tbsp olive oil
- 1 tsp dried or fresh thyme
- 1 small sprig of fresh rosemary
- Salt and pepper

Cooking Time: 50 min

Directions

1. Preheat your oven at 420F/215C. Line all the veggies in a baking sheet, drizzle with olive oil, and season with salt and pepper. Roast for 20-25 minutes.

2. Meanwhile, bring the vegetable stock to a boil. Add the roasted veggies and cook until softened for 20 minutes. Add the soy cream, thyme, and rosemary during the last 5 minutes of cooking.
3. Remove the rosemary from the soup and blend everything together using an immersion blender until smooth and creamy.
4. Season with extra salt and pepper if necessary and serve hot.

Nutritional Info (Per Serving)

Calories: 229kcal

Total Fat: 10.7

Saturated Fat: 1.4g

Cholesterol: 0mg

Carbs: 28.3g

Protein: 7.7g

Sodium: 1527mg

Fiber: 6.1g

Vitamins

A, C, K

Pasta & Shrimp Salad

A low fodmap recipe made with gluten-free pasta, olives, corn, and shrimps. Great for packed work lunches or light day meals.

Cuisine: International

Ingredients for 2-3 Servings

- 1 cup (100g) gluten-free penne pasta
- 4 cups (950ml) water
- ¾ cup (80g) cooked mini shrimps
- 1 tbsp sweet corn
- 6 black kalamata olives, halved
- 6 cherry tomatoes, halved
- 2 tbsp basil or coriander pesto sauce

Cooking Time: 20 min

Directions

1. Cook the gluten-free penne pasta in water for 15 minutes or according to package instructions. Drain and set aside.
2. Combine the pasta with all the veggies, shrimps toss, and add the basil pesto sauce. Stir and make sure the pasta and veggies are coated with the pesto sauce. Add shrimps.

3. Serve directly or keep in the fridge packed for up to 3 days.

Nutritional Info (Per Serving)

Calories: 249kcal

Total Fat: 11.2g

Saturated Fat: 1.3g

Cholesterol: 87mg

Carbs: 24.9g

Protein: 13.2g

Sodium: 675mg

Fiber: 4.6g

Vitamins

A, B12, K

Cream of Chicken Soup

A totally delicious and hearty soup, made with low FODMAP ingredients.

Cuisine: American

Ingredients for 4 Servings

- 4 skinless and boneless chicken thighs
- 2 large carrots, peeled and sliced
- 2 large potatoes, peeled and sliced
- 1 tbsp cornflour
- 5 cups (1182ml) chicken broth
- 1 cup (240ml) soy or almond cream
- 1 tbsp fresh chives, chopped
- 2 tbsp margarine
- Salt and pepper

Cooking Time: 45 min

Directions

1. Melt the margarine in a deep pan or medium pot, add the carrots and potatoes. Saute for 3-4 minutes.
2. Add the cornflour to the mix and stir with a spatula to coat the veggies. Add the chicken stock and thighs and bring to a boil over medium to low heat, for approx. 35-40 minutes. Add the soy

cream during the last two minutes of cooking and season with salt and pepper to taste.
3. Blend everything with an immersion blender or food processor until smooth and creamy.
4. Serve with the chives on top.

Nutritional Info (Per Serving)

Calories: 421kcal

Total Fat: 17.6g

Saturated Fat: 3.9g

Cholesterol: 93mg

Carbs: 44.4g

Protein: 22.8g

Sodium: 1153mg

Fiber: 4.3g

Vitamins

B6, A, C

Spicy Potato & Eggs Salad

A spicy version of the ordinary potato and egg salad, with a bit of bacon and mustard. A totally filling salad that will surely please everyone.

Cuisine: American

Ingredients for 4 Servings

- 3 large Yukon or russet potatoes, peeled and cubed
- 5 cups (1180ml) water
- 2 slices of bacon, cut into bits
- 4 large eggs
- 1 tbsp mustard
- 1 tbsp mayo
- 1 tsp paprika
- 1 tbsp red vinegar
- Salt and pepper

Cooking Time: 30 min

Directions

1. Boil the potatoes in salted water until softened but not too mushy.
2. Meanwhile, hard-boil the eggs for approx. 8 minutes. Rinse and keep them covered in ice-

cold water for a few minutes. Peel them off and cut them into small square pieces.
3. Cook the bacon bits in a pan for 2-3 minutes or until crispy.
4. Combine the mustard, mayo, and red vinegar in a mini bowl.
5. Combine the cooked potatoes with the eggs and add the creamy dressing mixture. Stir with a fork to gently mush everything together.
6. Season with salt, pepper, and dash paprika.
7. Finally, top with the bacon bits and serve.

Nutritional Info (Per Serving)

Calories: 343kcal

Total Fat: 11.2g

Saturated Fat: 1.9g

Cholesterol: 186mg

Carbs: 51.5g

Protein: 10.5g

Sodium: 1901mg

Fiber: 4g

Vitamins

B6, B1, Folate

Beef & Veggie Soup

A lovely soup recipe with ground beef, carrot, potatoes, and herbs that is good for all seasons.

Cuisine: International

Ingredients for 4 Servings

- 1 pound (450g) ground beef
- 5 cups (1180ml) beef broth
- 2 large russet or Yukon gold potatoes, peeled and cubed
- 2 carrots, peeled and sliced
- 2 tomatoes, peeled and cubed
- 15 green beans, trimmed and cut in half
- 1 tbsp Worcestershire sauce
- 1 tsp thyme
- 2 tbsp margarine
- Salt and pepper

Cooking Time: 45 min

Directions

1. Heat the margarine in a medium pot or large deep pan to melt.
2. Once melted, add the carrots, green beans, and potatoes. Saute for 3-4 minutes over medium heat and add the ground beef. Saute another 3-4

minutes until browned and season with salt, pepper, and thyme.
3. Add the beef broth and tomatoes and bring everything to a boil, for around 30 minutes or until the veggies are fully softened.
4. Finally, add the Worcestershire sauce. Season with extra salt and pepper if necessary and serve.

Nutritional Info (Per Serving)

Calories: 511kcal

Total Fat: 20.5g

Saturated Fat: 6.4g

Cholesterol: 100mg

Carbs: 39,5g

Protein: 41.3g

Sodium: 1893mg

Fiber: 3.6g

Vitamins

B12, A, B3

Seared Steak & Pepper Salad

A filling and delicious salad made with fresh or leftover strip steak, lettuce, and peppers in a mildly hot dressing.

Cuisine: American

Ingredients for 2 Servings

- 1 lb. (450g) New-Strip or flank steak, seared and sliced
- 1 large red bell pepper, thickly sliced
- 6 cherry tomatoes, halved
- 1 cup (40g) iceberg lettuce, roughly chopped
- 3 cups (75g) arugula leaves
- 1 tbsp white sesame seeds
- 3 tbsp olive oil
- 2 tbsp mustard
- Salt and pepper

Cooking Time: 15 min

Directions

1. Roasted the bell pepper slices with a drizzle of olive oil and salt/pepper in the oven's broiler (450F/230C) for 10 minutes.
2. In a small bowl, combine 2 tbsp olive oil and mustard to make your dressing.

3. Assemble your salad by mixing the arugula and lettuce leaves, the cherry tomatoes, and the red bell pepper first. Add the dressing and toss.
4. Add the steak slices on top of the salad and finally garnish with the sesame seeds.

Nutritional Info (Per Serving)

Calories: 505kcal

Total Fat: 28.2g

Saturated Fat: 7.1

Cholesterol: 136mg

Carbs: 9.8g

Protein: 52.3g

Sodium: 2722mg

Fiber: 3.4g

Vitamins

A, B6, C

Chicken Curry Noodle Soup

A favorite Indian dish becomes a hearty soup to warm and fill you up on cold days.

Cuisine: Indian

Ingredients for 4 Servings

- 3 boneless and skinless chicken thighs, thickly sliced
- 5 cups (1180ml) homemade chicken stock
- 1 (8 oz.) pack buckwheat or soba noodles
- 1 tbsp curry powder
- 1 tsp curry paste
- 1 tsp tomato paste
- 1 tbsp coriander leaves
- 2 tbsp vegetable oil
- Salt and pepper

Cooking Time: 20 min

Directions

1. Bring the chicken stock to a boil and add the noodles. Cook for 5-6 minutes over medium heat or according to package instructions(note: the noodles should not be fully cooked as they will cook a bit later with the remaining ingredients).

2. Meanwhile, add the vegetable oil to the pan, wait for it to become hot, and add the chicken thighs and the curry powder. Saute for 2-3 minutes.
3. Add the chicken to the cooked noodle soup and add the tomato and curry paste. Lower the heat to low and simmer for 10 minutes.
4. Serve warm with some coriander leaves for garnishing.

Nutritional Info (Per Serving)

Calories: 482kcal

Total Fat: 18.2g

Saturated Fat: 3.8g

Cholesterol: 80mg

Carbs: 50.7g

Protein: 31.7g

Sodium: 1741mg

Fiber: 1.4mg

Vitamins

B3, B6, K

Feta Cheese & Olives Quinoa Salad

A favorite Greek-style salad with quinoa, lettuce, olives, and peppers. Feta in this recipe is a low lactose/FODMAP cheese choice.

Cuisine: Greek

Ingredients for 4 Servings

- 8 oz. (225g) feta cheese, crumbled
- 1 cup (190g) quinoa, washed and drained
- 2 cups (475ml) water
- 5 kalamata olives, halved
- 5 cherry tomatoes, halved
- 1 medium head lettuce, roughly chopped
- 2 tbsp ACV vinegar
- 2 tbsp olive oil
- 1 tsp mint
- Salt and pepper

Cooking Time: 20 min

Directions

1. Cook the quinoa in boiling water for 15 minutes over medium to low heat. Cover and let sit for 10 minutes.

2. In a small bowl, combine the vinegar, olive oil, and salt/pepper. Assemble the salad by tossing the lettuce leaves, olives, and tomatoes together.
3. Add the cooked quinoa, toss and add the feta cheese. Add the dressing and garnish with a bit of dry mint on top.

Nutritional Info (Per Serving)

Calories: 381kcal

Total Fat: 22.1g

Saturated Fat: 9.7g

Cholesterol: 50mg

Carbs: 31.5g

Protein: 14.8g

Sodium: 571mg

Fiber: 3.8g

Vitamins

A, K, B2

Salmon Chowder

Rich and delicious salmon chowder with a hint of sweetness from sweet potatoes and coconut cream.

Cuisine: American

Ingredients for 5 Servings

- 1 pound (450g) unskinned salmon meat
- 1 cup (90g) chopped scallions (green parts only)
- 4 cups (946ml) unsweetened coconut milk
- 1 pound (450g) Yukon or russet potatoes, cubed
- 3 medium carrots, peeled and sliced
- 2 cups (475ml) fish broth
- 1 bay leaf
- 1 tsp thyme
- 2 tbsp margarine
- Salt and pepper

Cooking Time: 30 min

Directions

1. Heat the margarine in a deep pot or dutch oven to melt and add the scallion green bits. Saute until fragrant for 2 minutes.
2. Add the potatoes and carrots and saute for another minute. Add the fish broth, coconut milk, lay leaf, and thyme, and bring everything to a boil.

Once boiled, reduce the heat to low and simmer for 15 minutes.
3. Add the salmon to the pot and cook for another 5 minutes or until fish is cooked and opaque. Season with salt and pepper to taste and serve warm.

Nutritional Info (Per Serving)

Calories: 371kcal

Total Fat: 15.7g

Saturated Fat: 5.3

Cholesterol: 61mg

Carbs: 28.1g

Protein: 28,9g

Sodium: 765mg

Fiber: 4.3g

Vitamins

B6, D, B12

Nicoise Salad

A classic French salad with eggs, greens, and tomato. Great for any season.

Cuisine: French

Ingredients for 4 Servings

- 1 big romaine lettuce head, rinsed and roughly chopped
- 2 medium tomatoes, cut into quarters
- 2 large eggs
- 12 green beans, trimmed
- 3 cups (750ml) water
- 2 (5 oz.) tuna cans
- 1 tbsp dijon mustard
- 2 tbsp white vinegar
- 2 tbsp olive oil
- Salt and pepper

Cooking Time: 10 min

Directions

1. Hard-boil the eggs in boiling water for 7-8 minutes. Once boiled, leave in a chilled water bath for 2 minutes and peel. Cut each egg into quarters.

2. Meanwhile, cook the beans in boiling water for 10 minutes. Drain and set aside.
3. Combine the mustard, vinegar, and oil in a small bowl to make your dressing.
4. Assemble the salad by mixing in the lettuce, cooked greens, tuna, and tomatoes, and eggs. Add dressing and season with salt and pepper.

Nutritional Info (Per Serving)

Calories: 200kcal

Total Fat: 10.5g

Saturated Fat: 2.5g

Cholesterol: 121mg

Carbs: 8.9g

Protein: 19.4g

Sodium: 2013mg

Fiber: 4.5g

Vitamins

A, K, Folate

Healthy Vegan & Vegetarian Mains

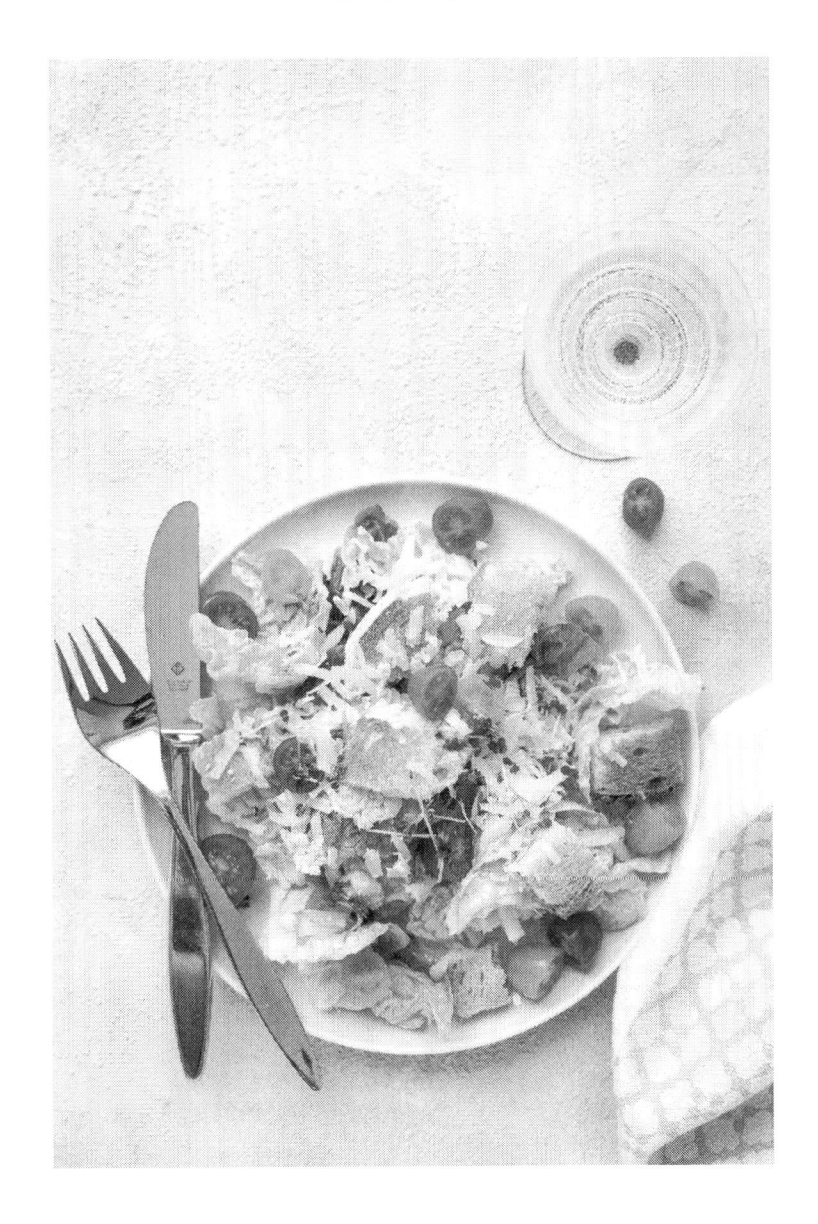

Veggie & Tofu Kebab

A colorful and delicious veggie and tofu kebab recipe with peppers, zucchini, and eggplants marinated in a delicious herb marinade.

Cuisine: International

Ingredients for 4 Servings

- 1 pack (14 oz./400g) firm tofu
- 1 red bell pepper, seeded and cut into squares
- 1 green bell pepper, seeded and cut into squares
- 1 large eggplant, cubed
- 1 large zucchini, thickly sliced into rounds
- 1 tsp chili flakes
- 1 tsp oregano
- 3 tbsp olive oil
- 2 tbsp vinegar
- 1 tbsp mustard
- Salt and pepper
- 7-8 thin wooden skewers
- Salad leaves (for garnishing)

Cooking Time: 20 min

Directions

1. Pinch the eggplant cubes with a fork and place them in a water bath to get rid of their bitterness. Soak the wooden skewers in water as well to prevent them from burning during cooking.
2. Prepare your marinade by mixing oil and vinegar with the herbs and salt/pepper to taste. Soak the cut veggies and the tofu cubes into the marinade and keep them in the fridge for at least an hour.
3. Preheat your oven's broiler to 450F/230C. Pass the tofu and veggie pieces interchangeably through the wooden skewers (around 8-10 pieces passed through each skewer).
4. Line a baking sheet with parchment paper and place the skewers on it. Bake the kebabs in the oven for approx. 18-20 minutes.
5. Serve ideally with a simple salad of choice e.g lettuce and tomatoes.

Nutritional Info (Per Serving)

Calories: 262 kcal

Total Fat: 17.8g

Saturated Fat: 2.5g

Cholesterol: 0g

Carbs: 15.6g

Protein: 15.1g

Sodium: 804mg

Fiber: 7.1g

Vitamins

A, C, B6

Veggies Frittata

A delicious brunch-lunch recipe made with low-fodmap veggies, eggs, and Mediterranean herbs.

Cuisine: Mediterranean

Ingredients for 4 Servings

- 8 large eggs, beaten
- 1 green bell pepper, sliced
- 1 yellow bell pepper, sliced
- 6 cherry tomatoes, halved
- 1 medium carrot, shredded
- 1 cup (80g) baby spinach leaves
- 1 (7oz./200g) pack feta cheese
- 1 tsp oregano
- 1 tsp thyme
- 2 tbsp olive oil
- Salt and pepper
- Greasing spray or oil

Cooking Time: 25 min

Directions

1. Heat the olive oil in a pan over medium to high heat and saute the bell peppers, carrot, and spinach for 2-3 minutes. Season with salt and pepper.

2. Mix the veggies with the eggs and feta cheese in a big bowl and add the thyme and oregano.
3. Grease the bottom of a 2-quart baking dish (round or rectangle) with oil or greasing spray. Pour the egg/veggie mixture into the dish and bake at 400F/200C for 15-18 minutes or until eggs are fully cooked.

Nutritional Info (Per Serving)

Calories: 413kcal

Total Fat: 30.7g

Saturated Fat: 14.4g

Cholesterol: 431mg

Carbs: 11.5g

Protein: 23.4g

Sodium: 815mg

Fiber: 1.8g

Vitamins

A, C, B2

Thai Pumpkin Noodles

A hearty recipe made with soy noodles, pumpkin puree, and a spicy Thai curry paste for lovers of spicy and ethnic flavors.

Cuisine: Thai/Fusion

Ingredients for 5 Servings

- 6 oz. (160g) buckwheat noodles
- 3 cups (710ml) homemade vegetable broth
- 1 cup (130g) pumpkin, cubed
- 2 medium carrots, diced
- 1 tbsp red curry paste
- 1 tsp cayenne pepper
- ¾ cup (180ml) unsweetened coconut milk
- 1 tsp fish sauce
- 1 tsp soy sauce
- 1 tbsp soybean oil
- Salt and pepper

Cooking Time: 25 min

Directions

1. Bring the vegetable broth to a boil and add the noodles. Cook for approx. 7-8 minutes or according to package instructions. Keep the noodles with the vegetable stock reserved.

2. In a separate deep pan, heat the oil and add the carrots and pumpkin cubes. Saute for 2-3 minutes and add enough water to cover and boil them. Simmer in medium to low heat for 20 minutes or until both are softened. Drain from the water and set aside.
3. Add a few tablespoons from the vegetable stock to the cooked pumpkin and carrots and blend well using an immersion blender.
4. Return the vegetables to the heat and add the curry paste, curry, cayenne, coconut milk, fish sauce, and soy sauce and bring to a boil. Finally, add the cooked noodles and the vegetable stock.
5. Season with salt and pepper to taste and serve warm.

Nutritional Info (Per Serving)

Calories: 299kcal

Total Fat: 23.5g

Saturated Fat: 10.1g

Cholesterol: 0g

Carbs: 17.6g

Protein: 9.6g

Sodium: 525mg

Fiber: 4.7g

Vitamins

A, B3, K

Sweet Potato Oven Fries & Salad

A crunchy and healthier variation of the ordinary french fries made with sweet potatoes and spices, roasted in the oven.

Cuisine: American

Ingredients for 4 Servings
- 3 medium sweet potatoes, peeled
- 1 tbsp cornstarch
- 1 tsp cayenne pepper
- 1 tbsp paprika
- 1 tsp thyme
- 2 tbsp parmesan cheese
- 3 tbsp olive oil
- Salt and pepper

For the salad
- 1 medium head of romaine lettuce, rinsed and roughly chopped
- 5 medium tomatoes, cut into quarters
- 1 medium parsnip, peeled and thinly sliced
- 1 tbsp pine nuts
- 2 tbsp olive oil
- 2 tbsp vinegar

- 1 tsp mustard
- Salt and pepper

Cooking Time: 40 min

Directions

1. Preheat your oven to 425F/220C. Cut the sweet potatoes with a sharp knife into thick sticks (the size of an ordinary french fry).
2. Add the potatoes to a bowl and toss in the spices and the cornstarch, making sure they are evenly coated.
3. Line a baking sheet with parchment paper and arrange the sweet potato fries, leaving around ½ inch or 1 cm space apart from each other. Sprinkle the olive oil.
4. Bake in the oven for 15 minutes on each side. During the last 5 minutes of cooking, sprinkle with the parmesan cheese.
5. Prepare your salad by combining the vegetables first and then saturate with the rest ingredients. Serve on the side once sweet potatoes are cooked.

Nutritional Info (Per Serving)

Calories: 324kcal

Total Fat: 18.9g

Saturated Fat: 2.9mg

Cholesterol: 0mg

Carbs: 40.7g

Protein: 6.3g

Sodium: 697mg

Fiber: 10.4g

Vitamins

A, K, Folate

Curry Quinoa Patties

A delicious patty/burger recipe with quinoa, veggies, and spices served in a homemade aioli (mayo)sauce.

Cuisine: American

Ingredients for 2 Servings

- ⅓ cup (80g) quinoa, washed and rinsed
- ¾ cup (200ml) homemade vegetable stock
- 1 large carrot, peeled and shredded
- ¼ cup/2 tbsp green scallions (green parts only), chopped
- 3 large eggs, beaten
- 4 tbsp cornstarch or almond flour
- 1 tsp paprika powder
- 1 tsp curry
- 1 tbsp vegetable oil
- Salt and pepper
- 3 tbsp olive oil

For the Aioli

- 2 tbsp mayo
- 1 tsp pepper
- 1 tsp garlic-infused oil
- 1 tsp lemon juice

Cooking Time: 25 min

Directions

1. Toast the quinoa with the oil in a pan or small deep pot for 2 minutes and add the vegetable stock. Cook covered for approx. 15 minutes or until quinoa has cooked and absorbed all the liquids.
2. Meanwhile, beat the eggs with the cornstarch in a big bowl and add the scallions, carrot, and spices. Once the quinoa is cooked, mix with the egg/veggie mixture. Season with salt and pepper. Let the mixture set in the fridge for 30-40 minutes then shape into round patties. Note: if they are sticky or hard to shape, dust your hands and the patties with extra cornflour.
3. Heat a pan with olive oil. Add the patties (3-4 at a time) and cook for approx. 3 minutes on each side.
4. Meanwhile, prepare your aioli by combining the mayo, infused oil, pepper, and lemon juice together.
5. Once the patties are ready, serve with the aioli on the side.

Nutritional Info (Per Serving)

Calories: 574kcal

Total Fat: 40.9g

Saturated Fat: 7.3g

Cholesterol: 282mg

Carbs: 43.4g

Protein: 9.2g

Sodium: 865mg

Fiber: 4.7g

Vitamins

A, C, K

Low Fodmap Pizza

A super easy and quick pizza made with low FODMAP veggies and cheese alternatives. It's vegetarian-friendly too.

Cuisine: Italian/Fusion

Ingredients for 2 Servings

- 2 large corn tortillas
- 1 cup (40g) spinach leaves
- 4 cherry tomatoes halved
- 1 large tomato, grated
- 1 tbsp sweet corn
- 3 tbsp mozzarella, grated
- 1 tbsp parmesan
- ½ tsp oregano
- ½ tsp basil
- Olive oil
- Salt and pepper

Cooking Time: 20 min

Directions

1. Preheat your oven to 400F/200C. Begin to assemble your pizza by layering one tortilla on top of each other so you get more volume as your crust/base.

2. Prepare your pizza sauce by combining the grated tomato with olive oil, basil, oregano, and salt/pepper to taste. Spread the pizza sauce evenly to the tortilla crust with a spoon or spatula (leave the crust edges uncovered).
3. Sprinkle with the mozzarella and parmesan cheeses and arrange the spinach leaves, tomatoes, and corn on top.
4. Bake for approx. 10 minutes. Once cooked, let sit for 5 minutes before cutting.

Nutritional Info (Per Serving)

Calories: 189kcal

Total Fat: 7.7g

Saturated Fat: 1.1g

Cholesterol: 5mg

Carbs: 19.7g

Protein: 12.3g

Sodium: 342mg

Fiber: 4.1g

Vitamins

A, K, C

Egg & Veggie Wraps

A lovely brunch/lunch recipe that is full of Tex-Mex flavors and nutrients to keep you satisfied and energized for hours.

Cuisine: Tex-Mex

Ingredients for 2 Servings
- 2 large corn tortillas
- 4 large eggs, beaten
- 1 red bell pepper, sliced
- ½ green red bell pepper, sliced
- 1 tsp chives
- 1 tsp cumin
- ½ tsp paprika
- ½ tsp coriander
- 2 tbsp vegetable oil
- Salt and pepper

Cooking Time: 10 min

Directions
1. Heat the oil in a medium pan and add the bell peppers. Saute for 2-3 minutes. Remove from the heat and set aside.
2. In the same pan, add the eggs, lower the heat, and scramble with a spatula. Once the eggs are

half-cooked, season with the herbs and spices and add salt and pepper to taste. Cook until eggs are set but not too dry.
3. Mix the eggs with the peppers and stuff your tortillas with the mixture. Fold in the edges and roll to make burrito-style packs.
4. Serve warm or keep in the fridge for up to 3 days wrapped with cling film.

Nutritional Info (Per Serving)

Calories: 226kcal

Total Fat: 14.8g

Saturated Fat: 14.8g

Cholesterol: 2.2g

Carbs: 15.1g

Protein: 9.5g

Sodium: 1288mg

Fiber: 2.4g

Vitamins

C, K, B2

Egg Shakshuka

A famous Middle-Eastern dish made with tomatoes, spices, and eggs. Very rich and filling for brunch or lunchtime.

Cuisine: Middle Eastern

Ingredients for 2 Servings

- 3 large tomatoes, peeled and grated
- 1 small carrot, peeled and shredded
- 4 small eggs
- ½ tsp cinnamon
- ½ tsp paprika
- ½ tsp cayenne pepper
- 2 tbsp olive oil
- 1 tbsp parsley
- Salt and pepper

Cooking Time: 20 min

Directions

1. Heat the olive oil in a pan and add the carrots. Saute for 2-3 minutes. Add the tomatoes and spices and season with salt and pepper to taste. Cook over medium heat for 10-12 minutes.
2. Crack the eggs (whole) over the tomato and carrot sauce and cover with a lid to trap the heat

and moisture. Cook until eggs are opaque and the yolk is cooked to your likes.
3. Garnish with the parsley leaves on top and season with extra salt and pepper if necessary to taste.

Nutritional Info (Per Serving)

Calories: 302kcal

Total Fat:21.5g

Saturated Fat:4.3g

Cholesterol:283g

Carbs: 17.2g

Protein:12.7g

Sodium:228g

Fiber: 5.2g

Vitamins

C, A, K

Basil & Spinach Pesto Risotto

A super delicious vegan risotto with homemade basil and spinach pesto sauce and corn.

Cuisine: Italian

Ingredients: for 4 Servings
- 1 ½ cup (300g) arborio rice
- 4 cups (1000ml) homemade vegetable stock
- 2 tbsp parmesan
- 1 tbsp sweet corn
- 1 tbsp pine nuts
- ½ cup (20g) spinach leaves
- 1 tbsp fresh basil leaves
- 2 tbsp olive oil
- 1 tbsp margarine
- Salt and pepper

Cooking Time: 20 min

Directions
1. Bring your vegetable stock to a boil and set it aside.
2. Toast the rice in 1 tbsp of olive oil in a deep pan or medium pot over medium heat.
3. Lower the heat and add the cups of stock to the rice gradually, around ½ cup at a time, stir, wait

for a couple of minutes and add the next part. Keep stirring every 1-2 minutes.
4. Prepare your pesto sauce by combining the spinach leaves, basil leaves, 1 tbsp olive oil, 1 tbsp parmesan cheese, pine nuts, and salt/pepper in a small food processor.
5. Once the risotto is nearly set (it should be al-dente and creamy), add the pesto sauce, the margarine, and the remaining parmesan cheese and stir well. Cook for another 2 minutes. Finally, add the corn.
6. Serve immediately.

Nutritional Info (Per Serving)

Calories: 250kcal

Total Fat: 19.1g

Saturated Fat: 3.3g

Cholesterol: 1mg

Carbs: 26.8g

Protein: 7.1g

Sodium: 986mg

Fiber: 9.4g

Vitamins

B1, B3, B6

Vegan Tofu Masala

A popular Indian dish made with a delicious masala spice mixture, tomatoes, and tofu. A great vegan choice for lunch or dinner.

Cuisine: Indian

Ingredients for 4 Servings

- 1 (4 oz./400g) pack firm tofu, cubed
- 1 (15oz./430g) can diced tomatoes
- 1 cup (40g) spinach, roughly chopped
- 1 ½ cup (370ml) unsweetened coconut milk
- 1 tbsp garam masala mix
- 1 tsp ginger powder
- 2 tbsp olive oil
- Salt and pepper

Cooking Time: 20 min

Directions

1. Heat the olive oil in a deep pan over medium heat and saute the spinach for a couple of minutes.
2. Add the diced tomatoes, coconut milk, masala mix, ginger, and salt and pepper to taste. Let cook for approx. 15 minutes over medium to low heat.
3. Add the coconut milk, stir, and add the tofu cubes. Cook everything for another 2-3 minutes.

4. Serve warm.

Nutritional Info (Per Serving)

Calories:415kcal

Total Fat:36g

Saturated Fat: 21.2g

Cholesterol: 0mg

Carbs:13.5g

Protein:17g

Sodium:1487mg

Fiber:6.3g

Vitamins

A, K, B1

Veggie "Meatballs" & Salad

A tasty vegetarian variation of ordinary meatballs, made with low-FODMAP veggies and a refreshing salad on the side.

Cuisine: International

Ingredients for 4 Servings
- 1 large zucchini, shredded
- 2 large potatoes shredded
- 1 large carrot, shredded
- 1 tsp thyme
- 1 tsp cinnamon
- 2 eggs
- 1 tbsp cornstarch
- Vegetable oil (for frying)
- 1 tbsp olive oil
- Salt and pepper

For the salad
- 2 cups (150g) romaine lettuce leaves
- 1 small carrot, shredded
- 2 tomatoes, cut into quarters
- ½ cup (120g) sweet corn
- 1 tbsp mustard
- 2 tbsp olive oil

- 1 tbsp vinegar
- Salt and pepper

Cooking Time: 20 min

Directions

1. Squeeze all the shredded veggies out to get rid of excess moisture.
2. Heat a deep pan with the olive oil and saute the veggies lightly for 2 minutes. Discard and set aside.
3. Transfer the veggies to a bowl and add the eggs, cornstarch, and spices. Mix well and shape the mixture with your hands, making small balls (a bit smaller than the size of a golf ball). Gently press them so they are cooked evenly later.
4. Heat the vegetable oil in a deep pan over medium to high heat. Once hot, add the meatballs (around 7-8 at a time). Cook until the balls have formed a golden-brown crust. Transfer into a dish lined with absorbing paper to absorb excess greasiness.
5. Prepare your salad by mixing in all the veggies first. Then, combine all the liquid dressing ingredients in a bowl and season with salt and pepper to taste. Pour the dressing over the salad just a few moments before serving the meatballs.
6. Serve the meatballs with the salad on the side.

Nutritional Info (Per Serving)

Calories: 393kcal

Total Fat: 19.1g

Saturated Fat: 3.3g

Cholesterol: 309mg

Carbs: 47.9g

Protein: 10.4g

Sodium: 318mg

Fiber: 7.1g

Vitamins

A, C, B12

Fish & Seafood

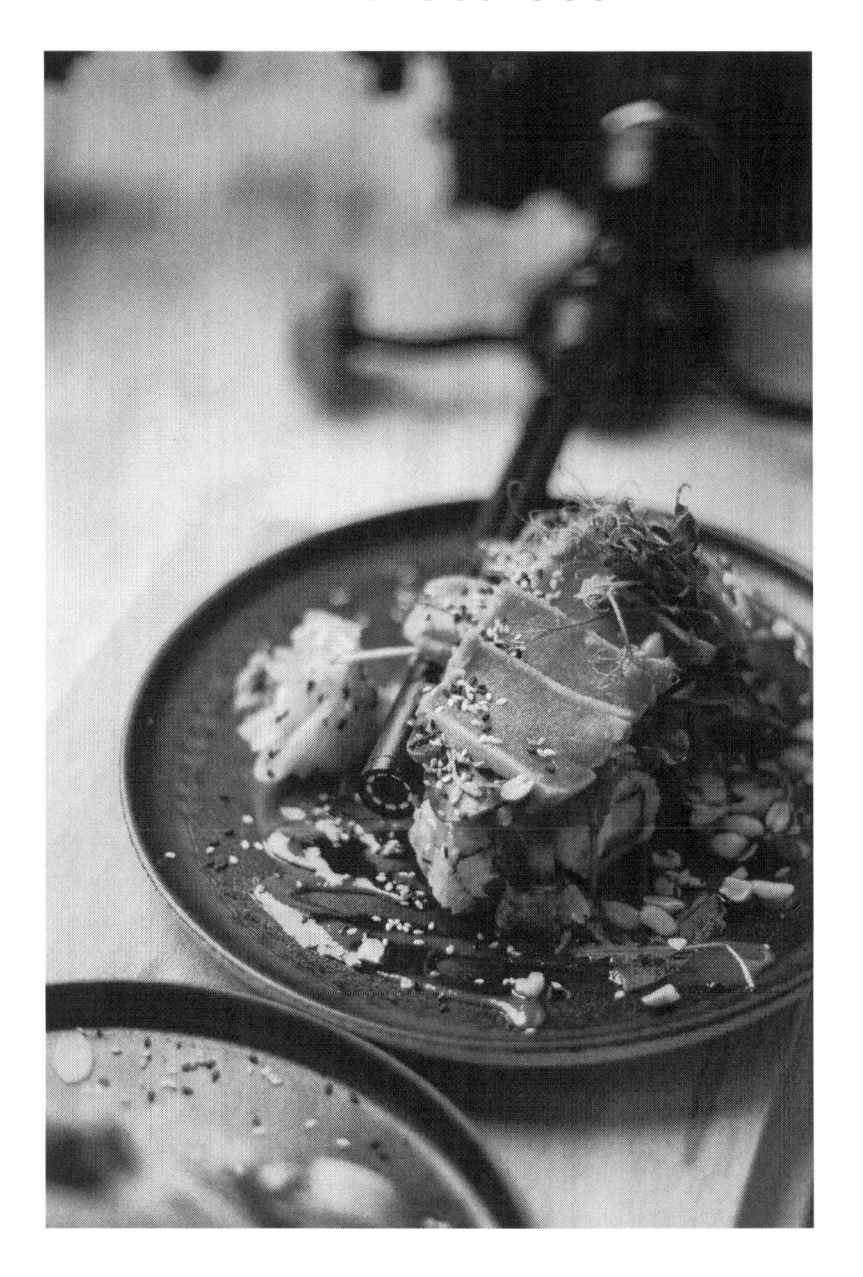

Mediterranean Fish Stew

A hearty fish stew inspired by the Mediterranean flavors of tomatoes, oregano, and capers. Great for weekend family lunch or dinner.

Cuisine: Mediterranean

Ingredients for 4 Servings

- 2 lbs (1kg) cod fillets, skinned and deboned
- 1 (15oz./425g) can tomatoes, diced
- 6 cherry tomatoes, halved
- 1 yellow bell pepper, sliced
- 1 red bell pepper, sliced
- 2 tbsp capers
- 2 tbsp white wine
- 3 cups (750ml) homemade vegetable broth
- 1 tbsp oregano
- 1 tbsp parsley leaves, chopped
- 2 tbsp olive oil
- Salt and pepper

Cooking Time: 40 min

Directions

1. Preheat your oven to 380F/190C.
2. Combine the vegetable broth and diced tomatoes in a deep casserole dish and add the fish and all

the remaining ingredients. Season with salt and pepper to taste.
3. Bake covered in the oven for 30 minutes. Once the 30 minutes are over, uncover and cook for another 10 minutes.
4. Serve warm.

Nutritional Info (Per Serving)

Calories: 266kcal

Total Fat: 8.2g

Saturated Fat: 1.2g

Cholesterol: 107mg

Carbs: 11.4g

Protein: 36.5g

Sodium:2078mg

Fiber: 3.2g

Vitamins

A, B12, C

Seafood Risotto

Delicious seafood risotto made with 3 kinds of seafood, combined ideally in a creamy risotto base.

Cuisine: Italian/Fusion

Ingredients for 4 Servings

- 1 ½ cup (240g) arborio rice, rinsed
- 12 small mussels, trimmed and cleaned
- 10 medium-size shrimps
- 2 oz. (50g) squid rings
- 5 cups (1200ml) fish stock
- 1 tbsp tomato paste
- 1 tbsp parmesan
- 1 tbsp margarine
- 2 tbsp olive oil
- 2 tbsp white wine
- Salt and pepper

Cooking Time: 25 min

Directions

1. Cut the heads off the shrimps and set them aside. Peel off the shrimps and leave the tail on.
2. Heat a deep pan with olive oil and add the shrimp heads. Saute for 2 minutes and add 3 cups of fish

stock and tomato paste. Bring the fish stock to a boil, remove the shrimp heads, and set aside.

3. In the same pan add the squid rings, mussels, shrimps (unheaded) and saute for around 2 minutes. Pour the wine and cook for another 2 minutes.
4. Add the rice, stir, lower the heat and gradually add the reserved fish stock in 4-5 parts, while stirring every time for a few seconds. Once the rice is nearly cooked (preferably a tad al-dente but creamy), add the parmesan cheese and margarine.
5. Season with extra salt and pepper if necessary and serve warm.

Nutritional Info (Per Serving)

Calories: 453kcal

Total Fat: 12.9g

Saturated Fat: 2.1g

Cholesterol: 61mg

Carbs: 62.1g

Protein: 19.5g

Sodium: 1213mg

Fiber:2.3g

Vitamins

B12, B3, C

Curry Calamari

A favorite Indian recipe with baby calamari rings cooked in spicy and creamy yellow curry sauce.

Cuisine: Indian

Ingredients for 4 Servings

- 10 mini calamari squids, washed (tentacles kept)
- 1 cup (240ml) unsweetened coconut milk
- 1 cup (240ml) vegetable or fish broth
- 1 tbsp curry powder
- 1 tsp yellow curry paste
- 1 tsp tomato paste
- 2 tbsp vegetable oil
- Salt and pepper

Cooking Time: 15 min

Directions

1. Heat the oil in a deep pan over medium fire and add the calamari squids. Saute for a couple of minutes.
2. Add the curry powder, curry paste, and tomato paste, and make sure the squids are covered evenly with the spices.
3. Add the unsweetened coconut milk and the veggie or fish broth and bring to a boil. Once

bubbles, reduce the heat to low and simmer everything for 10-12 minutes. Season with salt and pepper to taste.
4. Serve warm, preferably with brown or white rice.

Nutritional Info (Per Serving)

Calories: 230kcal

Total Fat: 11.1g

Saturated Fat: 2.7g

Cholesterol: 297mg

Carbs: 8.4g

Protein: 22.9g

Sodium: 277mg

Fiber: 1.2g

Vitamins

B12, B2

Pepper & Shrimps Pasta

A delicious pasta recipe with medium shrimps, bell peppers, tomatoes, and a touch of herbs. Great for lunch or dinner.

Cuisine: Italian

Ingredients for 5 Servings

- 1 lb (450g) gluten-free spaghetti pasta
- 5 cups (1200ml) water
- 10 medium shrimps, peeled and deveined
- 1 red bell pepper, sliced
- 3 large tomatoes, peeled and diced
- 1 tsp basil
- 1 tsp thyme
- 2 tbsp olive oil
- 1 tbsp parmesan cheese
- Salt and pepper

Cooking Time: 20 min

Directions

1. Cook the gluten-free pasta for 10 minutes in salted boiling water or according to package instructions. Drain and set aside.
2. Heat the olive oil in a deep pan and add the shrimps and peppers. Saute for 2 minutes or until

opaque (careful not to overcook). Add the diced tomatoes, and cook for another 3 minutes. Add the cooked pasta, toss, and season with the herbs and salt/pepper to taste.
3. Serve warm with the parmesan cheese on top.

Nutritional Info (Per Serving)

Calories: 200kcal

Total Fat: 6.5g

Saturated Fat: 1.1g

Cholesterol: 16mg

Carbs: 30.3g

Protein: 8.3g

Sodium: 1085mg

Fiber: 5.7g

Vitamins

A, C, E

Broiled Tilapia Fillets

A super quick and easy tilapia fillet recipe with mustard, herbs, and green scallions ready in just 20 minutes.

Cuisine: American/Fusion

Ingredients for 4 Servings

- 4 medium-to-large tilapia fish fillets, deboned
- 2 large scallion greens, chopped (green parts only)
- 3 tbsp mustard
- 1 tsp thyme
- A drizzle of olive oil
- Salt and pepper

Cooking Time: 20 min

Directions

1. Preheat your oven's broiler at 450F/230C.
2. Spread the mustard over the tilapia fillets and season with thyme and salt/pepper. Add the scallion green bits on top and drizzle with olive oil.
3. Line a baking sheet with parchment paper and transfer the tilapia fillets.
4. Cook for 10 minutes, open the oven and flip from the other side, cooking for another 8-10 minutes.

Nutritional Info (Per Serving)

Calories: 434kcal

Total Fat: 18.6g

Saturated Fat: 3.5g

Cholesterol: 156mg

Carbs: 4.1g

Protein: 63.6g

Sodium: 1720mg

Fiber: 1.4g

Vitamins

B12, D, K

Tuna & Sweet Potato Patties

A rich and delicious burger alternative made with canned tuna and sweet potatoes.

Cuisine: American

Ingredients for 4 Servings

- 2 (7-8 oz./200g each) cans of tuna, drained well
- 1 big sweet potato, peeled and shredded
- 1 large egg, cracked
- 1 tbsp cornstarch
- 1 tsp thyme
- 1 tsp paprika
- ½ tsp cinnamon powder
- ½ cup oil (120ml) for shallow frying
- Salt and pepper
- Lettuce leaves

Cooking Time: 10 min

Directions

1. Combine all the ingredients in a bowl. Place the mixture in the fridge to set for 30-40 minutes. Note: if it's too liquid, add more cornstarch.
2. Shape the mixture into 4 medium-sized patties (around 4" in diameter).

3. Heat the oil in a pan over medium to high heat and add the tuna patties. Shallow-fry for 3 minutes on each side.
4. Serve with a few lettuce leaves on the side.

Nutritional Info (Per Serving)

Calories: 476kcal

Total Fat: 30.1g

Saturated Fat: 3.5mg

Cholesterol: 103mg

Carbs: 19.8g

Protein: 33.4g

Sodium: 441mg

Fiber: 2.7g

Vitamins

B12, B6, C

Salmon & Mini Potatoes

A nice and tasty variation of the usual salmon and sweet potatoes, with mini potatoes and fresh herbs.

Cuisine: International

Ingredients for 4 Servings

- 4 (3-4oz/115g each) salmon fillets, skinned and deboned
- 10 mini potatoes, scrubbed and halved
- 1 tbsp fresh dill, chopped
- 1 tbsp fresh parsley, chopped
- 3 tbsp mustard
- 4 cherry tomatoes, halved
- ½ cup (120ml) olive oil
- 4 cups water
- Salt and pepper

Cooking Time: 30 min

Directions

1. Pre-boil the mini potatoes (hole) in boiling water for 10 minutes. Once boiled, cut in half (with the skin on).
2. Spread the mustard over the salmon fillets (making sure both sides are covered). Sprinkle

the dill and parsley on top and season generously with salt and pepper.
3. Line a square baking sheet with parchment paper and arrange the salmon fillets and potatoes on the side. Drizzle the potatoes with olive oil and add tomatoes.
4. Bake for 20 minutes at 390F/195C.

Nutritional Info (Per Serving)

Calories: 738kcal

Total Fat: 35.2g

Saturated Fat: 5.3g

Cholesterol: 66mg

Carbs: 77.6g

Protein: 30.1g

Sodium: 634mg

Fiber: 10.6g

Vitamins

C, B6, D

Tomato Fish Soup

Easy to cook soup with cod, tomato, carrots, peppers, and herbs.

Cuisine: Mediterranean

Ingredients for 4 Servings

- 4 medium cod fillets, deboned
- 8 jumbo shrimps, peeled and deveined
- 5 cups (1200ml) homemade vegetable or fish broth
- 1 (15 oz. can/425g) tomatoes, diced
- 2 red bell peppers, sliced
- 2 large carrots, sliced thinly
- 1 tsp tomato paste
- 2 tbsp red wine
- 2 tbsp olive oil
- 1 tbsp basil
- Salt and pepper

Cooking Time: 30 min

Directions

1. Heat the olive oil in a pot and add the carrots and peppers. Saute for 2-3 minutes. Finish with the wine.

2. Add the broth and diced tomatoes and bring to a boil. Reduce the heat to medium-low and boil the carrots and peppers for 15 minutes.
3. Add the codfish, shrimps, tomato paste, and basil, and cook over medium heat for another 10 minutes. Season with salt and pepper to taste.
4. Serve warm.

Nutritional Info (Per Serving)

Calories: 268kcal

Total Fat: 9.7g

Saturated Fat: 1.5g

Cholesterol: 146mg

Carbs: 8.1g

Protein: 36.6g

Sodium: 1546kcal

Fiber: 2.5g

Vitamins

B12, C, A

Fish Pie

A Low FODMAP version of the fish pie with carrots, potatoes, and cod or haddock with mashed potatoes.

Cuisine: English

Ingredients for 4 Servings

- 4 medium cod or haddock fillets, bones removed
- 1 cup (100g) mini shrimps, peeled and deveined
- 1 large carrot, cut into small cubes
- 4 medium potatoes, cut into small cubes
- 1 cup (240 ml) vegetable cream
- ½ cup (120ml) fish broth
- 1 tsp thyme
- 2 tbsp white wine
- 2 tbsp parmesan cheese
- 2 tbsp margarine
- 1 tsp cornstarch
- 2 tbsp vegetable oil
- 4 cups (1000ml) water
- Salt and pepper

Cooking Time: 55 min

Directions

1. Bring the water to a boil and add the potatoes and carrots. Boil until softened (around 15 minutes).
2. Add the potatoes and carrots to a deep pan with the vegetable oil, saute for 1-2 minutes and add the wine. Let evaporate. Keep half of the potatoes aside in a dish.
3. Add the veggie cream, corn starch, and the fish broth to the pan and cook until sauce has thickened (approx. 7-8 minutes).
4. Smash the reserved potatoes with a smasher and add the margarine and salt/pepper to taste. Stir in the parmesan cheese.
5. Combine the veggie sauce with the fish and the shrimps in a casserole dish. Season with the thyme and top with a layer of mashed potatoes (use a spoon or spatula to even everything out).
6. Bake in the oven at 400F/200C for 25-30 minutes.

Nutritional Info (Per Serving)

Calories: 268kcal

Total Fat: 9.7g

Saturated Fat: 1.5g

Cholesterol: 146mg

Carbs: 8.1g

Protein: 36.6g

Sodium: 1546mg

Fiber: 2.5g

Vitamins

B12, A, C

Soy Glazed Salmon & Sesame

A favorite Asian-style recipe that looks fancy but is actually very easy to make and ready in under 20 minutes.

Cuisine: Asian

Ingredients for 2 Servings

- 2 (3-4oz. each) salmon fillets, skinned and deboned
- 3 tbsp soy sauce
- 1 tsp maple syrup
- ½ tsp ginger powder
- 1 tbsp rice vinegar
- 1 tbsp white sesame seeds
- 1 tbsp vegetable oil
- Salt and pepper

Cooking Time: 18 min

Directions

1. Preheat your oven at 400F/200C.
2. In a small bowl, combine the soy sauce, maple syrup, rice vinegar, ginger powder, and vegetable oil to make your marinade.

3. Season your salmon fillets with salt and pepper and soak them in the marinade. Keep in the fridge for at least 1 hour.
4. Bake the salmon fillets in the oven for 15-18 minutes.
5. Serve with the sesame seeds on top.

Nutritional Info (Per Serving)

Calories:640kcal

Total Fat:28.5g

Saturated Fat: 5.5g

Cholesterol:293mg

Carbs:8.7g

Protein:82.2g

Sodium:1725mg

Fiber:1g

Vitamins

B12, B3, D

Poultry & Meat

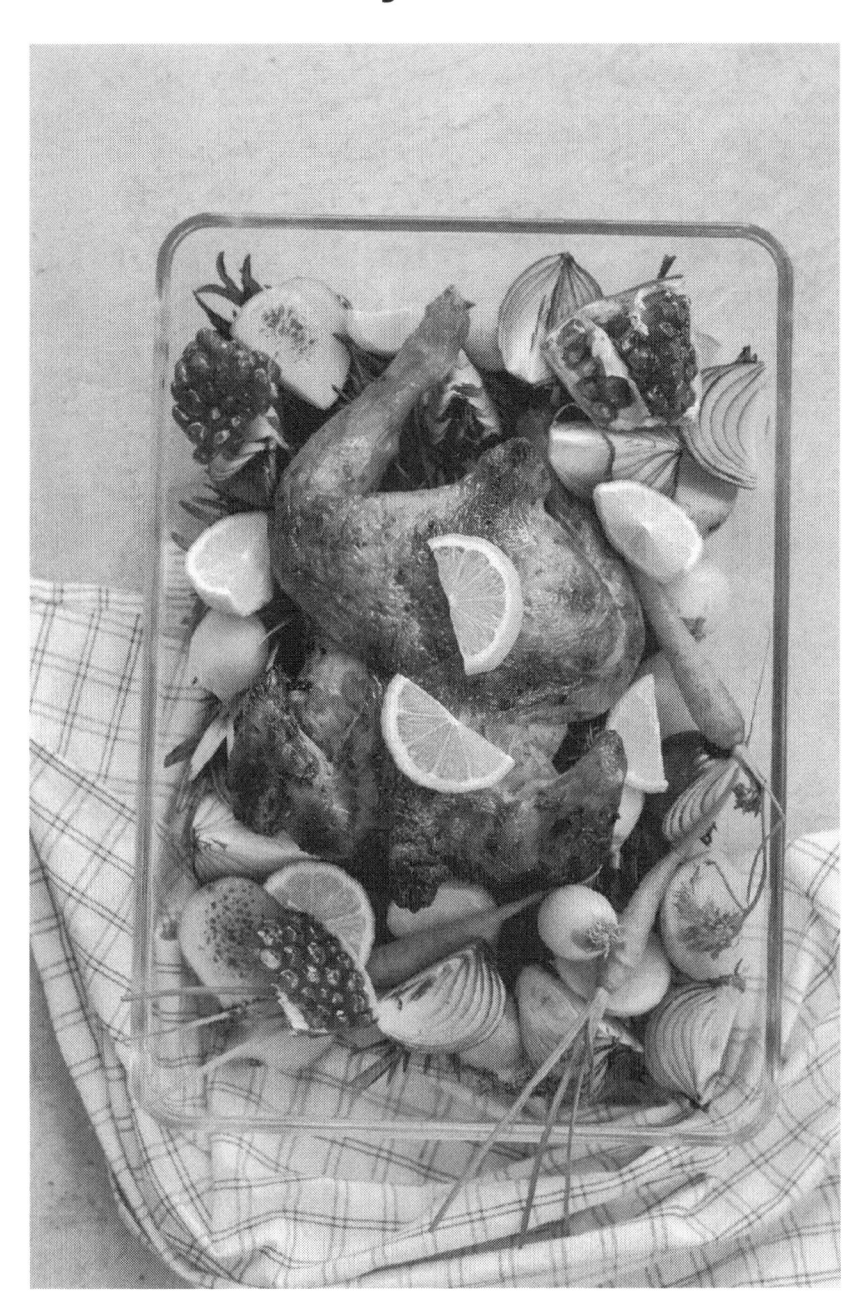

Chicken Piccata

A low-FODMAP and gluten-free version of chicken piccata, with a light breading of cornstarch, eggs, and a zesty lemon-caper sauce.

Cuisine: French

Ingredients for 4 Servings

- 6 chicken thighs, skinned and deboned
- 2 tbsp cornstarch or almond flour
- 2 large lemons, juiced
- 1 cup (240 ml) vegetable broth
- 2 large eggs, beaten
- 1 tbsp capers
- ½ cup (120 ml) vegetable oil
- Salt and pepper
- 2 cups (400g) cooked brown rice

Cooking Time: 20 min

Directions

1. Keep the corn starch or almond flour and beaten eggs in two separate bowls. Season both with salt and pepper.
2. Dip the chicken thighs in the egg wash first and then the flour. Make sure all their sides are coated well with the egg and flour breading.

3. Heat a deep pan with the vegetable oil over medium heat and shallow fry the chicken thighs until golden brown on the outside and white/greyish on the inside (they should be juicy but no pink inside). Remove excess oil from the pan (leave only a few tablespoons) and add the lemon, vegetable broth, and capers. Reduce the heat and cook until the sauce has thickened, for around 10 minutes.
4. Serve with the rice on the side.

Nutritional Info (Per Serving)

Calories: 746kcal

Total Fat: 50.7g

Saturated Fat: 19.4g

Cholesterol: 311mg

Carbs: 30.5g

Protein: 41.1g

Sodium: 520mg

Fiber: 2.2g

Vitamins

B6, B3, C

Low Fodmap Beef Stew

A Low Fodmap version of beef stew with carrots, potatoes, and herbs, slowly cooked in a slow cooker or Dutch oven.

Cuisine: English

Ingredients for 5 Servings

- 2 lbs(1kg) beef chuck cubes, for stew
- 2 medium carrots, sliced
- 2 medium potatoes, cubed
- 1 (15oz./425g) can diced tomatoes
- 2 cups (480ml) beef broth
- 2 tbsp red wine
- 1 bay leaf
- 1 tbsp thyme
- ½ cup (120ml) vegetable oil
- 1 tbsp Worcestershire sauce
- Salt and pepper

Cooking Time: 3 – 3 ½ hours

Directions

1. Heat the vegetable oil in a deep pan and brown the beef cubes over high heat until browned (approx. 1-2 minutes on each side) but not fully cooked. Remove from the heat and add the

potatoes and carrots. Saute for 2-3 minutes and add back the beef cubes. Pour the wine and let evaporate.

2. Transfer the seared beef and veggies to a slow cooker or dutch oven and add the beef broth, diced tomatoes, bay leaf, spices, and Worcestershire sauce. Season with salt and pepper to taste.
3. If you are using a slow cooker, cook on medium heat for approx. 3 hours. If you are using a dutch oven, cook at 300F/150C for 3 hours and 15 minutes.

Nutritional Info (Per Serving)

Calories: 525 kcal

Total Fat: 27.1g

Saturated Fat: 19.3g

Cholesterol: 153mg

Carbs: 28.4g

Protein: 42.1g

Sodium: 1943mg

Fiber: 4.1g

Vitamins

B3, B6, B12

Pesto Chicken Kebabs

An easy and quick kebab/skewer recipe made with chicken breasts and homemade low-FODMAP pesto.

Cuisine: Mediterranean

Ingredients for 4 Servings

- 3 large chicken breasts, skinned and deboned
- 2 tbsp fresh basil leaves
- 2 tbsp coriander leaves
- 3 tbsp olive oil
- 1 tbsp pine nuts
- 1 tbsp parmesan cheese
- ½ tsp lemon zest
- Salt and pepper
- Greasing spray

Cooking Time: 20 min

Directions

1. Combine the herbs, pine nuts, olive oil, lemon zest, and parmesan cheese in a small food processor until you end up with an oily green paste.

2. Cut the chicken breasts into equal size cubes and pass through wooden skewers, around 6-7 pieces through each skewer.
3. Brush the pesto mixture onto the chicken kebabs and season with salt and pepper.
4. Grease a grilling pan with greasing spray and cook the chicken kebabs for around 3 minutes on each side. They should look char-grilled on the outside but not pink on the inside.

Nutritional Info (Per Serving)

Calories: 515kcal

Total Fat: 220.8g

Saturated Fat: 4.1g

Cholesterol: 249mg

Carbs: 1.3g

Protein: 81.3g

Sodium: 1592mg

Fiber: 0.2g

Vitamins

B3, C, B6

Pork Chops in Bacon Mustard Sauce & Mashed Potatoes

A rich pork chop recipe with creamy low-FODMAP mustard, maple, and bacon sauce.

Cuisine: International

Ingredients for 5 Servings

- 5 medium bone-in pork chops
- 4 large potatoes, peeled and cubed
- 3 cups (710ml) vegetable broth
- 2 tbsp dijon mustard
- 2 thin strips of bacon, chopped
- 1 cup (240 ml) soy or almond cream
- 2 tbsp margarine
- 1 tbsp chives, chopped
- 2 tbsp olive oil
- 4 cups (1000ml) water
- Salt and pepper

Cooking Time: 50 min

Directions

1. Heat the olive oil in a pan and sear the pork chops for 2 minutes on each side. Take off the heat.
2. Add the vegetable broth and mustard and bring to a boil. Lower the heat and return the pork

chops to the pan. Cook over medium to low heat for approx. 45 minutes.

3. Meanwhile, boil the potatoes in a separate pot filled with 4 cups of water for approx. 20-25 minutes or until totally soft. Once cooked, remove from the heat and drain. Add the margarine and season with chives and salt/pepper to taste.
4. Once the pork chops are nearly done, add to the pan the soy or almond cream and the bacon bits and cook for another 5 minutes.
5. Serve the pork chops with the sauce and mashed potatoes on the side.

Nutritional Info (Per Serving)

Calories: 730kcal

Total Fat: 33.2g

Saturated Fat: 8.1g

Cholesterol: 132mg

Carbs: 60.2g

Protein: 47.2g

Sodium: 2234mg

Fiber: 7g

Vitamins

B1, B3, B6

Lamb & Spinach Curry

A rich curry recipe with lamb, tomatoes, and spinach in a creamy textured sauce.

Cuisine: Indian

Ingredients for 4 Servings

- 6 lamb chops, excess fat trimmed
- 1 ½ cups (45g) spinach leaves
- 1 tbsp curry powder
- 1 tsp cayenne powder
- 2 cups (480ml) unsweetened coconut milk
- 1 cup (240ml) vegetable broth
- 2 large tomatoes, diced
- 1 tbsp tomato paste
- 1 tsp ginger powder
- 2 tbsp vegetable oil
- Salt and pepper

Cooking Time: 40 min

Directions

1. Heat the oil in a pan and sear the lamb chops for approx. 1-2 minutes on each side. Remove from the heat and set aside.
2. In the same pan, add the tomatoes and spinach and saute for 2 minutes. Add the vegetable broth,

curry powder, ginger, cayenne pepper, tomato paste, and bring to a boil. Once boiled, reduce the heat and add the lamb chops. Simmer for 30 minutes. Add the coconut milk and season with salt and pepper to taste.
3. Cook for another 5 minutes and serve warm.

Nutritional Info (Per Serving)

Calories: 261kcal

Total Fat: 15.6g

Saturated Fat: 5.1g

Cholesterol: 54mg

Carbs: 13.8g

Protein: 18.1g

Sodium: 978mg

Fiber: 2.7g

Vitamins

A, K, B12

Beef & Broccoli

A favorite Chinese dish with beef strips and broccoli in a light soy sauce mixture and sesame seeds for extra crunch.

Cuisine: Asia

Ingredients for 2 Servings

- 1 large head of broccoli, cut into small florets
- 2 medium (4-5oz. each) beef tenderloin or strip steaks, cut into thin strips
- 2 tbsp soy sauce
- 3 tbsp sesame oil
- ½ cup (120ml) oyster sauce
- ½ cup (120ml) homemade beef stock
- 1 tbsp sesame seeds
- 1 tsp cornstarch
- Salt and pepper

Cooking Time: 20 min

Directions

1. Heat 2 tbsp of the sesame oil in a pan and add the broccoli. Saute for 7-8 minutes over medium heat. Remove and set aside
2. Add the beef strips to the pan with the remaining sesame oil and saute for 2 minutes.

3. Return the broccoli to the pan with the beef and add the soy sauce, oyster sauce, and beef stock. Add the cornstarch and cook over medium heat until the mixture thickens or forms small bubbles. Season with salt and pepper to taste.
4. Serve with sesame seeds on top.

Nutritional Info (Per Serving)

Calories: 669kcal

Total Fat: 33.8g

Saturated Fat: 6.5g

Cholesterol: 120mg

Carbs: 36.1g

Protein: 61.6g

Sodium: 2671mg

Fiber: 9.1g

Vitamins

C, K, B6

Chicken & Pork Meatloaf

A satisfying chicken and pork meatloaf with eggs and carrots on the side. A perfect dinner recipe.

Cuisine: American/Fusion

Ingredients for 8 Servings

- 1 lb (500g) ground pork
- 1 lb (500g) lean ground chicken (from chicken breasts)
- 2 large potatoes, peeled and cubed
- 5 medium eggs
- 1 medium carrot, shredded
- 1 small zucchini, shredded
- 1 tsp paprika
- 1 tbsp mustard
- 2 tbsp tomato juice
- 3 tbsp oats
- ½ cup (120ml) olive oil
- Salt and pepper

Cooking Time: 45 min

Directions

1. Preheat your oven to 390F/195C.

2. Combine 2 eggs, tomato juice, and oats in a big bowl and add the ground pork and chicken to the mix.
3. Heat 1-2 tbsp olive oil and saute the shredded carrot and zucchini for 1-2 minutes.
4. Add to the ground meat mixture and add the remaining spices and mustard. Season with salt and pepper.
5. Hard boil 3 eggs for 7-8 minutes. Once boiled, keep in a bowl with ice-cold water for at least 5 minutes before peeling.
6. Line a baking sheet with parchment paper on top, take half of the meatloaf mixture and shape it into a large rectangle (around 8" long). Make three shallow holes across its length (make sure to leave some ground meat underneath) and place one egg at each hole. Take the remaining meatloaf mixture and cover the eggs and the sides, shaping well with your hands.
7. In a separate bowl, coat the potato cubes generously with olive oil and season with salt and pepper to taste.
8. Place the potatoes around the meatloaf and pour the remaining oil on top of everything.
9. Bake for 40 minutes.

Nutritional Info (Per Serving)

Calories: 455kcal

Total Fat: 25.3g

Saturated Fat: 6.9g

Cholesterol: 211mg

Carbs: 18.9g

Protein: 37.5g

Sodium: 978mg

Fiber: 2.8g

Vitamins

B6, A, B3

Sausage, Peppers & Eggs

A quick and easy sausage and pepper fry with cracked eggs and a light tomato sauce. Perfect for any time of the day.

Cuisine: Mediterranean

Ingredients for 4 Servings

- 2 links Spicy Italian or Greek sausage, thickly sliced
- 2 green bell peppers, diced
- 1 red bell pepper, diced
- 4 large eggs
- 2 cups (480ml) diced tomatoes
- 1 tbsp tomato paste
- 1 tsp oregano
- 1 tbsp red wine
- 2 tbsp olive oil
- Salt and pepper

Cooking Time: 20 min

Directions

1. Heat the olive oil in a pan and add the sausage and peppers. Saute for 2 minutes and add the red wine. Wait a few seconds and add the diced tomatoes and tomato paste. Season with spices

and salt/pepper to taste. Cook over medium heat for 15 minutes.
2. Crack the eggs on top of the mixture and scrabble slightly with a spatula. Cover and let cook until eggs are set (5 minutes extra).
3. Serve.

Nutritional Info (Per Serving)

Calories: 218kcal

Total Fat: 15.1g

Saturated Fat: 3.9g

Cholesterol: 197mg

Carbs: 8.4g

Protein: 11g

Sodium: 257mg

Fiber: 1.7g

Vitamins

A, C

Sweet Potato, Chicken & Veggies Bake

A delicious and filling bake recipe with sweet potato, various veggies, and chicken. Great for family or guest feasts.

Cuisine: International

Ingredients for 6 Servings
- 2 large sweet potatoes, peeled and cubed
- 3 chicken breasts (no skin), cubed
- 4 large eggs, beaten
- 2 tbsp soy cream
- 1 large carrot, sliced
- 1 large zucchini, sliced
- 1 tbsp thyme
- 1 tsp oregano
- 4 oz. (150g) feta cheese, crumbled
- 3 tbsp olive oil
- Salt and pepper
- 4 cups (1000ml) water

Cooking Time: 50 min

Directions

1. Pre-boil the carrots and sweet potatoes in salted water for 10 minutes. Drain and set aside. Preheat the oven at 400F/200C.
2. Grease generously the bottom of a 3-quart baking dish with oil and add the carrots, sweet potatoes, zucchini, and chicken pieces. Season with the spices.
3. In a small separate bowl, beat together the eggs and soy cream. Pour the mixture over the veggies and make sure to coat them well. Top with the crumbled feta cheese.
4. Bake everything for 40 minutes.

Nutritional Info (Per Serving)

Calories: 225kcal

Total Fat: 15.3g

Saturated Fat: 3.9g

Cholesterol: 199mg

Carbs: 8.2g

Protein: 14.5g

Sodium: 901mg

Fiber: 1.7g

Vitamins

C, A, B12

Spicy Lamb Meatballs & Pumpkin Mush

A spicy meatball recipe made with ground lamb and herbs, accompanied by a delicious pumpkin mush.

Cuisine: International

Ingredients for 4 Servings

- 1 lb (450g) ground lean lamb
- 2 cups (400g) pumpkin, peeled and diced
- 1 egg, beaten
- 2 tbsp fresh coriander, chopped
- 1 tbsp fresh parsley, chopped
- 1 tsp chili flakes
- 1 tsp lemon zest
- 1 tbsp oats
- 2 tbsp olive oil
- 2 tbsp margarine
- 2 tsp cinnamon
- 4 cups (1000ml) water
- Salt and pepper

Cooking Time: 40 min

Directions

1. Combine the ground lamb with olive oil, egg, oats parsley, coriander, chili flakes, and lemon zest. Season with salt and pepper. Let the mixture sit in the fridge for 20 minutes.
2. Preheat the oven at 390F/195C and line a wide baking sheet with parchment paper on top. Shape the ground lamb mixture into small balls with your hands (around 15-17 balls). Bake in the oven for 30 minutes.
3. Meanwhile, boil the pumpkin in salted water for 20-25 minutes or until completely soft. Drain well, mash with a masher or blend in the food processor with margarine and cinnamon. Season with salt and pepper to taste.
4. Serve the meatballs with the pumpkin puree on the side.

Nutritional Info (Per Serving)

Calories: 440kcal

Total Fat: 37.2g

Saturated Fat: 13.6g

Cholesterol: 124mg

Carbs: 6.4g

Protein: 21.8g

Sodium: 1293mg

Fiber: 1.5g

Vitamins

A, K, C

Sesame Chicken Bites

A delicious breaded chicken bites recipe made with a low-FODMAP breading and a light sweet and sour sauce.

Cuisine: Asian

Ingredients for 4 Servings

- 3 large chicken breasts, skinned and cut into cubes
- 2 tbsp cornstarch
- 2 tbsp oat flour
- 3 whole eggs, beaten
- 1 tsp Chinese 5-spice mix
- 2 tbsp soy sauce
- 1 tbsp sesame seeds
- 1 cup (240ml) pineapple juice
- 1 tbsp apple cider vinegar
- 1 tbsp tomato paste
- 1 tbsp brown sugar
- 1 tbsp oyster sauce
- Salt and pepper
- Oil (for frying)

Cooking Time: 25 min

Directions

1. Combine the cornstarch, oat flour, and sesame seeds in a bowl and keep the beaten eggs in another bowl.
2. Coat the chicken bites with the soy sauce and dip into the eggs first, then the cornstarch/oat flour/sesame mixture. Make sure all their sides are coated.
3. Heat your oil in a pan and add the breaded chicken bites. Fry for 5-6 minutes or until golden brown and crispy. Remove from the heat and set aside.
4. In the same pan, take off excess oil, and add the pineapple juice, oyster sauce, tomato paste, and brown sugar and bring to a boil. Season with salt and pepper to taste.
5. Return the chicken bites to the heat, add 5-spice mix and vinegar, and cook for another 5 minutes.
6. Serve with their sauce.

Nutritional Info (Per Serving)

Calories: 533kcal

Total Fat: 26.3g

Saturated Fat: 7.3g

Cholesterol: 262mg

Carbs: 19.6g

Protein: 51.4g

Sodium: 1015mg

Fiber: 0.9g

Vitamins

B3, B6, B12

Stuffed Beef Peppers

A quick and easy recipe made with bell peppers stuffed with a delicious mixture of ground beef and veggies.

Cuisine: American

Ingredients for 4 Servings

- 2 large green bell peppers, halved and seeds removed
- 1 lb. (500g) ground beef (80%lean)
- 1 small carrot, shredded
- 1 tbsp tomato paste
- 2 tbsp sweet corn
- ½ cup (120ml) tomato juice
- 1 tsp cayenne pepper
- ½ cup (122g) cheddar cheese, shredded
- 2 tbsp vegetable oil
- Salt and pepper

Cooking Time: 30 min

Directions

1. Heat the oil in a pan and brown the beef. Add the carrots and veggies, stir and add the tomato paste and the tomato juice. Cook everything for

7-8 minutes on low heat. Season with cayenne pepper and salt/pepper to taste.
2. Stuff the 4 pepper halves with the ground beef mixture and top with the cheddar cheese (around 1 tbsp for each halve).
3. Bake at 400F/200C for 20 minutes.

Nutritional Info (Per Serving)

Calories: 434kcal

Total Fat: 34.5g

Saturated Fat: 12.4g

Cholesterol: 96mg

Carbs: 6.7g

Protein: 23.9g

Sodium: 1242mg

Fiber: 1.8g

Vitamins

B12, A, C

Pork Stir-Fry & Noodles

An Asian-style pork stir-fry with a soy sauce base, peppers, spring onion greens, and buckwheat noodles.

Cuisine: Asian

Ingredients for 4 Servings

- 1 medium (1 ½ lbs/700g) pork tenderloin, excess fat removed
- 2 red bell peppers, cut into strips
- 1 (10oz./300g) pack, soba buckwheat noodles
- 2 spring onions, green parts only
- 1 cup (240ml) beef or chicken broth
- 1 tsp Chinese 5-spice mix
- 2 tbsp soy sauce
- 1 tbsp rice vinegar
- 1 tbsp tomato paste
- 1 tsp chili flakes
- 4 cups (1000ml) water
- 2 tbsp sesame oil
- Salt and pepper

Cooking Time: 25 min

Directions

1. Cook the buckwheat noodles in boiling water for 7-8 minutes or according to package instructions. Drain and set aside.
2. Cut the pork into thick strips. Heat the sesame oil in a deep pan or wok and add the pork strips, spices, scallion greens, and peppers, and stir-fry for 3 minutes. Add the soy sauce, Chinese spice mix, rice vinegar, beef (or chicken) broth, and tomato paste and cook until the sauce bubbles.
3. Serve warm.

Nutritional Info (Per Serving)

Calories: 611kcal

Total Fat: 17.4g

Saturated Fat: 3.9g

Cholesterol: 117mg

Carbs: 58.7g

Protein: 57.1g

Sodium: 1592mg

Fiber: 0.9g

Vitamins

B1, B6, B3

Greek-Style Chicken Thighs

An easy and delicious chicken thigh recipe with Greek herbs and a balsamic vinegar marinade.

Cuisine: Greek/Fusion

Ingredients for 4 Servings

- 8 chicken thighs, skinless and deboned
- 1 tbsp oregano
- 1 tsp thyme
- ½ cup (120ml) tbsp Greek ouzo or sweet white wine
- 1 tsp lemon zest
- 1 lemon, squeezed
- ¼ cup (60ml) olive oil
- Greasing spray
- Salt and pepper

Cooking Time: 25 min

Directions

1. Combine all the liquid ingredients and herbs in a bowl. Add the chicken thighs, coat well with the marinade, and season with salt and pepper and marinate in the fridge for at least an hour.
2. Heat a grilling pan and sear the chicken thighs for 1-2 minutes on each side.

3. Transfer into a greased baking sheet and bake in your oven's broiler (450F/230C) for another 15 minutes.

Nutritional Info (Per Serving)

Calories: 798kcal

Total Fat: 63.3g

Saturated Fat: 15.3g

Cholesterol: 292mg

Carbs: 5.6g

Protein: 49.9g

Sodium: 1408g

Fiber: 0.7g

Vitamins

B3, B6, B12

Italian Meatballs & Zucchini Noodles

A low-FODMAP and healthier version of the famous Italian meatballs with zucchini noodles in place of ordinary pasta.

Cuisine: Italian

Ingredients for 4 Servings

- 1 ½ lb (700g) ground beef
- 2 large zucchinis, made into zoodles with a spiralizer
- 1 tbsp Italian seasoning
- 2 tbsp fresh basil, chopped
- 1 tbsp tomato paste
- 1 tsp paprika
- 2 cups (400g) diced tomatoes (fresh or canned)
- 2 tbsp olive oil
- 2 tbsp pesto sauce
- 2 tbsp parmesan cheese
- Salt and pepper

Cooking Time: 30 min

Directions

1. Combine the ground beef with herbs, tomato paste, 1 tbsp pesto sauce, basil, and 1 tbsp olive oil. Season with salt and pepper.
2. Line a wide baking sheet with parchment paper and shape the beef mixture into 14-16 small balls with your hands.
3. Bake in the oven at 400F/200C. Meanwhile, heat 1 tbsp of olive oil in a pan and add the zucchini noodles. Add the remaining pesto sauce and cook for 2-3 minutes. Remove from the heat and set aside.
4. In the same pan and the tomatoes and bring to a boil. Season with salt and pepper to taste.
5. Once everything is cooked, serve the zoodles with tomato sauce, meatballs, and parmesan cheese on top.

Nutritional Info (Per Serving)
Calories: 538kcal
Total Fat: 35.4g
Saturated Fat: 11.8g
Cholesterol: 152mg
Carbs: 7.7g
Protein: 45.3g
Sodium: 1681mg
Fiber: 3.2g

Vitamins

B12, B3, B1

Easy Turkey Roast

The easiest and quickest way to roast a turkey, made with just 6 ingredients.

Cuisine: American

Ingredients for 6 Servings

- 1 small turkey (around 8 lbs/3.5Kg)
- 2 large carrots, sliced
- 2 tbsp thyme
- 2 sprigs rosemary
- ½ cup (120ml) olive oil
- 5 cups (1200ml) chicken stock
- Salt and pepper

Cooking Time: 2 ½ hour

Directions

1. Pre-boil the turkey in boiling stock for 20 minutes, over medium heat (use a cover). Reserve half of the chicken stock. Preheat your oven to 350F/175C.
2. Transfer the turkey to a baking tray and drizzle generously with the olive oil and season with thyme, salt, and pepper. Place the rosemary springs and carrot below the turkey or on the

sides. Pour the reserved stock on the sides of the baking dish/tray.

3. Bake the turkey and carrots for 2 hours covered and 15 minutes uncovered.

Nutritional Info (Per Serving)

Calories: 953kcal

Total Fat: 491.1g

Saturated Fat: 10.5g

Cholesterol: 381mg

Carbs: 2.5g

Protein: 118.7g

Sodium: 1628mg

Fiber: 0.4g

Vitamins

B3, B6, B12

Low Fodmap BBQ Pork Chops

A low-FODMAP variation of BBQ pork chops, with a homemade BBQ sauce. Perfect for grilling or broiling.

Cuisine: American

Ingredients for 4 Servings

- 4 large bone-in pork chops
- 1 cup (220ml) tomato puree
- 1 tbsp maple syrup
- 1 tbsp smoked paprika
- 1 tsp liquid smoke
- 1 tbsp vegetable oil
- Salt and pepper

Cooking Time: 30 min

Directions

1. Combine the tomato puree, maple syrup, liquid smoke, vegetable oil, and smoked paprika in a saucepan and bring to a boil. Once the mixture boils, reduce the heat and simmer for 15 minutes.
2. Brush the BBQ sauce generously over the pork chops, making sure all sides are coated well with the sauce. Add salt and pepper.

3. Grill the pork chops on a grilling pan or BBQ rack for 5-6 minutes on each side. Alternatively, you can broil them at 450F/230C for 25 minutes.

Nutritional Info (Per Serving)

Calories: 404kcal

Total Fat: 21.5g

Saturated Fat: 6.1g

Cholesterol: 132,g

Carbs: 11g

Protein: 41.6g

Sodium: 730mg

Fiber: 2.1g

Vitamins

B3, B6, A

Chicken Stuffed with Spinach & Ricotta Cheese

A restaurant-grade and easy-to-make recipe with chicken thighs stuffed with ricotta cheese and spinach. Served with boiled cauliflower on the side.

Cuisine: Italian

Ingredients for 4 Servings

- 8 chicken thighs (boneless and skinless)
- 1 large head cauliflower, cut into small florets
- ¾ cup (190g) ricotta cheese
- 1 tbsp parmesan, grated
- 2 cups (60g) spinach leaves, roughly chopped
- 1 cup (240ml) concentrated tomato juice
- 1 tbsp dried or fresh basil
- 1 tsp pesto sauce
- 2 tbsp olive oil
- Salt and pepper

Cooking Time: 40 min

Directions

1. Pound the chicken thighs lightly and season with salt and pepper on both sides.

2. Heat 1 tbsp of olive oil and saute the spinach leaves for 2 minutes. Drain excess juices/moisture.
3. Combine the spinach, ricotta cheese, parmesan, and pesto in a medium mixing bowl with a fork.
4. Slash the chicken thighs with a knife and pat them flat. Spoon off one part of the spinach/ricotta cheese mixture in the center of each chicken thigh and roll carefully, making sure it doesn't stick out of the sides. Secure the ends with a toothpick.
5. Bake the chicken thighs at 380/190C for 30 minutes. Meanwhile, prepare your tomato sauce and cauliflower. For the tomato sauce, heat 1 tbsp of olive oil and add the tomato juice and basil leaves. Season with salt and pepper to taste. Cook over medium heat for 15 minutes.
6. In another pot, cook the cauliflower in boiling water for 20 minutes.
7. Once the chicken thighs are ready, pour the tomato sauce on top and serve the cauliflower on the side.

Nutritional Info (Per Serving)

Calories: 832kcal

Total Fat: 62.7g

Saturated Fat: 18.4g

Cholesterol: 316mg

Carbs: 8.6g

Protein: 57.1g

Sodium: 405mg

Fiber: 2.8g

Vitamins

K, B3, B6

Pumpkin Beef Chili

A lovely sweet twist to the famous beef chili with pumpkin and sweet corn. Great for family or guest dinners.

Cuisine: American

Ingredients for 5 Servings
- 1 lb (500-600g) ground beef
- 1 cup (240ml) beef broth
- 1 cup (116g) pumpkin, diced
- 1 red chili pepper, sliced
- 1 cup (240ml) tomato juice
- ½ cup (85g) sweet corn
- 1 tbsp tomato paste
- 1 tsp chili flakes
- 3 tbsp vegetable oil
- Salt and pepper

Cooking Time: 40 min

Directions
1. Heat the vegetable oil in a pan and saute the ground beef with the pumpkin for 2-3 minutes. Season with salt, pepper, and chili flakes.

2. Add the corn, tomatoes, and beef broth and bring to a boil. Once boiled reduce the heat to low and simmer for 30 minutes.
3. Add the chili pepper during the last 2 minutes of cooking. Serve warm.

Nutritional Info (Per Serving)

Calories: 442kcal

Total Fat: 30.3g

Saturated Fat: 7.3g

Cholesterol: 80mg

Carbs: 11.4g

Protein: 33.3g

Sodium: 1326mg

Fiber: 3g

Vitamins

B3, B12, C

Peanut Butter Chicken

A simple Asian-style chicken dish with creamy peanut butter and coconut cream sauce.

Cuisine: Asian

Ingredients for 6 Servings

- 1 whole chicken, cut into 6-8 bone-in pieces
- 2 tbsp unsweetened peanut butter
- 1 ½ cup (368ml) unsweetened coconut cream
- 3 tbsp sesame or olive oil
- 1 ½ cup (300g) basmati rice
- 3 cups vegetable broth
- Salt and pepper

Cooking Time: 30 min

Directions

1. Heat the oil in a deep pan and sear the chicken pieces for 2-3 minutes on each side. Season with salt and pepper.
2. Combine the peanut butter and coconut milk in a bowl and add to the chicken. Cook over medium to low heat for 30 minutes.
3. Meanwhile, prepare your rice by boiling the broth first and then adding the basmati rice. Cook for approx. 15 minutes.

4. Serve the chicken with the sauce and rice on the side.

Nutritional Info (Per Serving)

Calories: 549kcal

Total Fat: 38.9g

Saturated Fat: 21.8g

Cholesterol: 103mg

Carbs: 21.4g

Protein: 38.8g

Sodium: 1060mg

Fiber: 2.1g

Vitamins

B3, B6, Folate

Sweet Snacks & Desserts

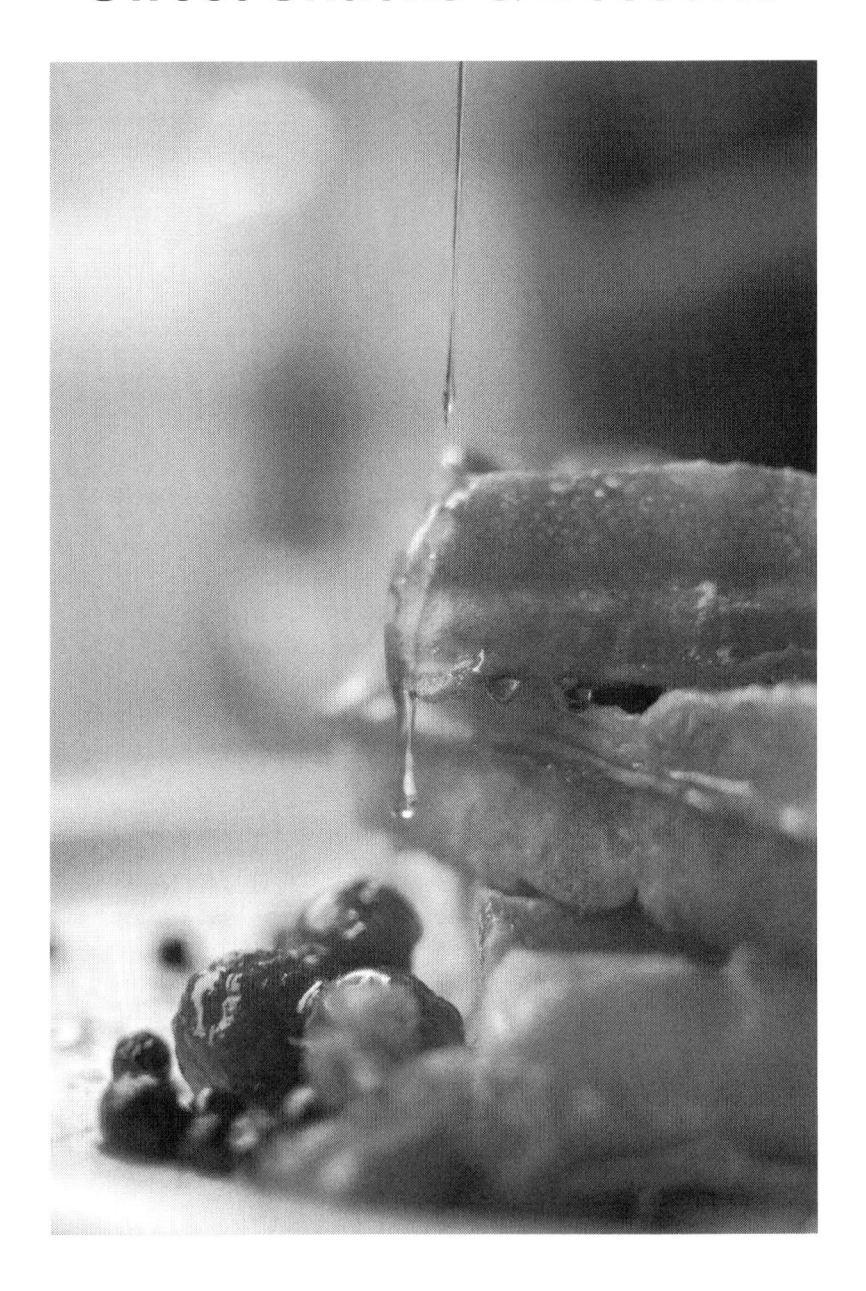

Low FODMAP Carrot Energy Balls

A delicious carrot energy ball recipe with rolled oats and shredded carrots; it tastes a bit like carrot cake with a hint of pumpkin spices but much healthier.

Cuisine: International

Ingredients for 10 Servings (10 balls)
- ½ cup (60g) rolled oats
- 2 medium carrots, shredded
- 1 tbsp unsweetened peanut butter
- 1 tbsp coconut oil
- 2 tbsp flax seeds
- ½ tsp cinnamon
- ½ tsp ginger

Cooking Time: 10 min

Directions
1. Process everything in the food processor until you end up with a thick paste.
2. Shape the mixture with your hands into 10 small bite-size balls.
3. Let sit in the fridge for at least one hour before serving.

Nutritional Info (Per Serving)

Calories: 44kcal

Total Fat: 2.9g

Saturated Fat: 1.3g

Cholesterol: 0g

Carbs: 5.1g

Protein: 1.4g

Sodium: 36mg

Fiber: 1.4g

Vitamins

A, B1, E

Chocolate Brownies

A family and guest favorite dessert made with gluten-free flour and coconut oil, offering a guilt-free sweet pleasure.

Cuisine: American

Ingredients for 40 small brownies
- ½ cup (75g) almond or oat flour
- 1 cup (2 sticks) unsalted butter
- 8 oz (225g) dark chocolate, chopped
- 1 cup (200g) white sugar
- 4 large eggs, at room temperature
- 1 tsp baking powder
- 1 tbsp vanilla extract
- 1 tsp ground coffee
- ⅔ cup (75g) toasted pecans, chopped

Cooking Time: 35 min

Directions
1. Mix the flour, coffee, sugar, and baking powder in a bowl and set aside.
2. Melt the chocolate and butter in a double-boiler (Ben-Marie) method.
3. In a separate bowl, beat the eggs with the vanilla extract.

4. Mix the melted chocolate mixture with the flour mixture and slowly incorporate the eggs.
5. Transfer the mixture into a 9X13" rectangle baking pan and press with a spatula to even and smooth everything out.
6. Sprinkle the chopped pecans over half of the brownie batter and press gently with a spoon.
7. Bake at 350F/175C for 30 minutes. The brownies are done when you insert a toothpick and it comes out clean. Take off the oven and let cool for 15 minutes.
8. Make 8X5 lines to cut into 40 squares. If not served immediately, keep stored for up to 5 days at room temperature.

Nutritional Info (Per Brownie)

Calories: 95kcal

Total Fat: 7.2g

Saturated Fat: 3.5g

Cholesterol: 25mg

Carbs: 6.2g

Protein: 1.2g

Sodium: 6mg

Fiber: 0.9g

Vitamins

A, B12

Low FODMAP Lemon Cake

A decadent lemon cake recipe with a white lemon frosting. This is both low-FODMAP and gluten-free and so it's ideal for people with gluten intolerance as well.

Cuisine: International

Ingredients for 10 Servings

- 1 cup (225g) softened butter or margarine
- 2 cups (250g) gluten-free flour e.g. almond
- 4 eggs, beaten
- ½ cup (120ml) almond milk
- 1 tbsp lemon zest
- 1 tbsp lemon juice
- Greasing spray

For the frosting

- 1 ½ cup (250g) powdered sugar
- 3 tbsp lemon juice
- 1/4 cup(50g) softened butter

Cooking Time: 50 min

Directions

1. Preheat the oven to 350F/175C. Grease a long cake tin with greasing spray and line with parchment paper (covering all sides).

2. In a bowl, combine the dry cake ingredients first and then mix gradually the remaining liquid ingredients.
3. Pour the cake batter in the tin and bake for 45-50 minutes or until you insert a toothpick and it comes out clean.
4. During the last 10 minutes of baking, prepare your frosting. Heat the butter/margarine in a saucepan and add the lemon juice. Slowly mix in the sugar (around 5 parts) while whisking continuously. Cook until you end up with a heavy liquid syrup.
5. Leave the cake to sit and chill at room temperature for 10 minutes. Pour the lemon frosting on top, starting from the center and then outwards.
6. Cut a few pieces and serve.

Nutritional Info (Per Serving)

Calories: 294kcal

Total Fat: 24.6g

Saturated Fat: 9.5g

Cholesterol: 97mg

Carbs: 16.9g

Protein: 2.6g

Sodium: 77mg

Fiber: 0.1g

Vitamins

A, K, E

Easy No-Bake Cookies

If you don't have the time and resources to use your oven, these easy no-bake cookies are perfect for a quick-no-bake sweet snack.

Cuisine: International

Ingredients for 55-60 cookies

- 2 cups (400g) white sugar
- ½ cup (120ml) unsweetened almond milk
- ½ cup (4 tbsp) unsalted butter or vegetable shortening
- 3 tbsp cocoa powder
- 3 cups (600g) rolled oats
- 1 cup (240g) unsweetened peanut butter
- 1 tsp vanilla extract

Cooking Time: 40 min

Directions

1. Line a baking sheet with parchment paper.
2. In a medium saucepan mix in the milk, butter, sugar, vanilla extract, and cocoa and bring to a boil. Let boil for 1 minute.
3. Combine the mixture with the rolled oats and peanut butter.

4. Drop the cookie batter with a large spoon onto the baking tray (drop around 55-60 pieces).
5. Let the mixture sit and harden for 30 minutes or keep in the fridge for up to 40 minutes before serving.

Nutritional Info (Per Cookie)

Calories: 91kcal

Total Fat: 4.6g

Saturated Fat: 1.5g

Cholesterol: 5mg

Carbs: 10.6g

Protein: 2.6g

Sodium: 12mg

Fiber: 1.3g

Vitamins

B1, B3

Low FODMAP Pumpkin Pie Mousse

A super quick and easy to prepare pumpkin pie mousse with pumpkin puree, coconut cream, and nuts for extra crunch on the top.

Cuisine: International

Ingredients for 2 Servings
- ½ cup (120g) pumpkin puree
- ¼ cup (60ml) unsweetened coconut cream
- 2 tbsp brown sugar
- 2 tbsp raw peanut butter
- 1 tsp cinnamon
- 1 tsp vanilla extract
- 1 semi-ripe banana
- 2 tbsp chopped almonds

Cooking Time: 5 min

Directions
1. Combine all the ingredients (except for the chopped almonds) in a food processor until creamy and smooth.
2. Place the mixture into 2 dessert glasses or mason jars and top with the chopped almonds.

3. Chill in the fridge for at least 2 hours before serving.

Nutritional Info (Per Serving)

Calories: 253kcal

Total Fat: 14.1g

Saturated Fat: 9.8g

Cholesterol: 0mg

Carbs: 30.8g

Protein: 3.4g

Sodium: 243mg

Fiber: 3.5g

Vitamins

A, B6, C

Fruit Salad

A zesty fruit salad combining the exotic fruity flavors of pineapple, kiwi, and bananas.

Cuisine: International

Ingredients for 6 Servings

- 1 large pineapple, peeled and cubed
- 2 semi-ripe bananas, sliced
- 3 kiwis, cut into squares
- 3 cups (720ml) orange juice
- 1 tbsp maple syrup

Cooking Time: 10 min

Directions

1. Combine all the ingredients in a large salad bowl.
2. Chill in the fridge for at least one hour before serving.

Nutritional Info (Per Serving)

Calories: 262kcal

Total Fat: 2.7g

Saturated Fat: 0.4g

Cholesterol: 0mg

Carbs: 61.9g

Protein: 2.9g

Sodium: 21mg
Fiber: 5.1g

Vitamins

A, C, E

Stovetop Sweet Popcorn

A delicious pick-me-up snack and dessert made with popcorn and salted brown sugar.

Cuisine: American

Ingredients for 10 Servings

- ½ cup dry corn kernels
- ⅓ cup (50g) brown sugar
- 1 tsp sea salt
- 3 tbsp coconut oil
- ⅓ cup (80ml) vegetable oil

Cooking Time: 15 min

Directions

1. Heat the vegetable oil in a deep pot over medium heat and add the corn kernels. Cover with the lid, toss every 2 minutes and cook until nearly all corn kernels have popped.
2. Meanwhile, heat the coconut oil in a pan and add the brown sugar and sea salt. Reduce the heat to low and cook until you end up with a thick grainy syrup.
3. Once the popcorn is ready add the brown sugar mixture and toss well to combine and serve.

Nutritional Info (Per Serving)

Calories: 155kcal

Total Fat: 11.6g

Saturated Fat: 9.4g

Cholesterol: 0mg

Carbs: 13.2g

Protein: 0.7g

Sodium: 237mg

Fiber: 0.6g

Vitamins

B6, B1

Carrot Cake

A decadent carrot cake recipe with a gluten-free flour base and a creamy cheese frosting on top.

Cuisine: American

Ingredients for 10 Servings

- 1 ⅓ cup (180g) almond or oat flour
- 1 cup (175g) brown sugar
- 2 large carrots, grated
- 3 whole eggs, beaten
- 2 tbsp baking powder
- 1 tsp nutmeg
- 1 tsp cinnamon powder
- 1 tsp vanilla extract

For the frosting

- 7 oz. (200g) cream cheese
- 2 cups (250g) icing sugar
- 2 tbsp unsalted butter

Cooking Time: 50 min

Directions

1. Preheat the oven at 350F/175C and line a long cake tin with parchment paper.

2. Mix all the dry cake ingredients in a large mixing bowl and add the carrots, eggs, and vanilla extract.
3. Pour the cake batter into the cake tin and even out with a spatula. Bake for 45-50 minutes or until you insert a toothpick and it comes out clean.
4. Prepare your cream cheese frosting by melting the butter and then adding the icing sugar and cream cheese. Let cook until sugar is dissolved.
5. Let the cake cool at room temperature for 10 minutes and spread the cream cheese frosting on top.

Nutritional Info (Per Serving)

Calories: 276kcal

Total Fat: 9.8g

Saturated Fat: 5.2g

Cholesterol: 70mg

Carbs: 42.9g

Protein: 5.3g

Sodium: 122mg

Fiber: 1.6g

Vitamins

A, B2, B1

Chocolate, Peanut Butter & Roasted Bananas

A super easy and delicious kid-friendly dessert with just 4 ingredients. So easy that even your kids can make.

Cuisine: American

Ingredients for 12 Servings
- 2 large semi-ripe bananas, thickly sliced
- ½ cup (70g) chocolate shaves
- 3 tbsp unsweetened raw peanut butter
- 2 tbsp maple syrup

Cooking Time: 10 min

Directions
1. Preheat your oven to 350F/175C. Line a baking tray and arrange the banana slices, leaving a few inches of spice apart from each other.
2. Spread a thin layer of peanut butter onto each banana slice and sprinkle with the chocolate shaves. Bake for 8 minutes.
3. Once ready, let cool at room temperature for 15 minutes and serve with maple syrup. You may

also enjoy these chilled (at least 1 hour in the fridge).

Nutritional Info (Per Serving)

Calories: 75kcal

Total Fat: 0.9g

Saturated Fat: 0.2g

Cholesterol: 0mg

Carbs:16.5g

Protein: 0.7g

Sodium: 70mg

Fiber: 1g

Vitamins

B6, C

Easy Matcha Pudding

A super easy and quick pudding recipe with green matcha powder, soy yogurt, and coconut cream.

Cuisine: Asian

Ingredients for 2 Servings

- 1 ½ cup (370g) plain soy or almond yogurt
- ½ cup (120ml) coconut cream
- 1 tbsp matcha green powder, sifted
- 1 tbsp gelatin powder.
- 2 tbsp maple syrup
- ½ tsp lemon zest

Cooking time: 5 min

Directions

1. Combine all the ingredients in a food blender and process until smooth and creamy.
2. Transfer the mixture into 2 dessert glasses or mason jars and chill in the fridge for at least 3 hours before serving.

Nutritional Info (Per Serving)

Calories: 369kcal

Total Fat: 23.8g

Saturated Fat: 18.8g

Cholesterol: 0mg
Carbs: 35.3g
Protein: 6.8g
Sodium: 33mg
Fiber: 2.1g

Vitamins

D, C, B2

3-Week Meal Plan
1st Week:

	Breakfast	Lunch	Snack	Dinner
MON	Strawberry &Kiwi Smoothie	Mustard Bacon Pork Chops	2-3 pieces choco banana bites	Sweet Potato Oven Fries
TUE	Egg & Veggie Wrap	Pasta & Shrimp Salad	2 slices carrot cake	Lamb meatballs & pumpkin
WED	Quinoa Jar	Peanut Butter Chicken	1 cup sweet pop-corn	Spicy tomato & pepper soup
THU	Green Smoothie	Pork Stir-Fry	2 chocolate brownies	Low FODMAP pizza
FRI	Banana -Almond Pancakes	Grilled Chicken & Berry Salad	1 serving green matcha pudding	Sweet Potato & Veggies Bake
SAT	Stuffed Sweet Potatoes	Turkey Roast	4 no-bake cookies	Chicken/Curry Noodle Soup
SUN	Chocolate & Coffee Smoothie	Fish Pie	2 slices lemon cake	Beef Stew

2nd Week:

	Breakfast	Lunch	Snack	Dinner
MON	Quiche breakfast bake	BBQ pork chops	Pumpkin Pie Mousse	East Spinach Soup
TUE	Potato & zucchini hash browns	Seafood risotto	1 cup sweet popcorn	Sausage, Pepper & Eggs
WED	Strawberry & kiwi smoothie	Greek chicken thighs	1 cup fruit salad	Pepper & Shrimps Pasta
THU	Quinoa jar	Curried calamari	Banana & peanut butter bites	Carrot & Parsnip Soup
FRI	Spinach & Eggs Omelette	Tuna & sweet potato patties	2 slices lemon cake	Sesame Chicken Bites
SAT	Cornbread Waffles	Vegan tofu masala	2 pieces choco brownies	Pumpkin Beef Chili
SUN	Green Detox Smoothie	Chicken & pork meatloaf	2 slices carrot cake	Salmon & Baked Potatoes

3rd week:

	Breakfast	Lunch	Snack	Dinner
MON	Egg Shakshuka	Italian Meatballs	1 cup fruit salad	Tomato fish soup
TUE	Pineapple & carrot smoothie	Spinach & lamb curry	2 pieces brownies	Curried quinoa patties
WED	Sage Sausage	Pesto chicken kebabs	Carrot energy balls	Broiled tilapia fillets
THU	Salmon scrambled eggs	Veggie meatballs & salad	1 serving matcha pudding	Stuffed beef peppers
FRI	Green detox smoothie	Stuffed chicken & spinach	4 no-bake cookies	Veggies frittata or salmon chowder
SAT	Chocolate Breakfast Bowl	Beef & broccoli	1 cup sweet popcorn	Spinach & pesto risotto
SUN	Quinoa Breakfast Bowl	Mediterranean fish stew	2 slices lemon cake	Cream of chicken soup

Conclusion

If you are experiencing IBS symptoms and want to eliminate any foods that trigger your symptoms, the low FODMAP diet is the best choice you can make for treating your condition, at least on a temporary basis. It may be a tad restricting but as you can see, there are multiple recipes and meal ideas to explore and we have gathered 80 of the best recipes here. Most of these are quick and easy to make and so you can dedicate a couple of hours 2X a week and prepare all your weekly meals in advance or simply go fresh if you have time to spend in the kitchen every day. Once the 3 weeks have passed, you can lax your diet and re-introduce higher-FODMAP foods gradually. We suggest during the re-introduction phase that you introduce FODMAPs from one particular group at a time (each week) e.g dairy products one week, higher FODMAP fruits the next so you know which FODMAPs seem to affect your system the worse and avoid them during the final adjustment phase.

Keep in mind that the low-FODMAP diet is a lifestyle choice, not another restricting weight-loss diet where you limit calories so you can lose weight. However, if your secondary goal is to lose weight as well, you may consume smaller portions in each daily meal and consume up to 1800 calories daily (depending on your body type) so you can lose some weight while controlling your IBS symptoms. It's also best to consult an expert nutritionist in this case so you can reach all your goals without any risky experimentation on your own.

Good luck on your low-FODMAP diet journey.

Written by: Albert Simon
Copyright © 2021
All rights reserved.

All Rights Reserved. No part of this publication or the information in it may be quoted from or reproduced in any form by means such as printing, scanning, photocopying, or otherwise without prior written permission of the copyright holder.

Disclaimer and Terms of Use: Effort has been made to ensure that the information in this book is accurate and complete, however, the author and the publisher do not warrant the accuracy of the information, text, and graphics contained within the book due to the rapidly changing nature of science, research, known and unknown facts, and internet. The Author and the publisher do not hold any responsibility for errors, omissions, or contrary interpretation of the subject matter herein. This book is presented solely for motivational and informational purposes only.

Made in the USA
Las Vegas, NV
28 October 2023